Pediatric Intensive Care – Practice and Research

Pediatric Intensive Care – Practice and Research

Guest Editors

Martin E. G. Blohm
Dominique Singer

MDPI

Basel • Beijing • Wuhan • Barcelona • Belgrade • Novi Sad • Cluj • Manchester

Guest Editors
Martin E. G. Blohm
Neonatology and Paediatric Intensive Care Medicine
Altona Children's Hospital (AKK)
Hamburg
Germany

Dominique Singer
Neonatology and Pediatric Critical Care Medicine
University Medical Center Eppendorf (UKE)
Hamburg
Germany

Editorial Office
MDPI AG
Grosspeteranlage 5
4052 Basel, Switzerland

This is a reprint of the Special Issue, published open access by the journal *Children* (ISSN 2227-9067), freely accessible at: https://www.mdpi.com/journal/children/special_issues/Intensive_Care.

For citation purposes, cite each article independently as indicated on the article page online and as indicated below:

Lastname, A.A.; Lastname, B.B. Article Title. *Journal Name* **Year**, *Volume Number*, Page Range.

ISBN 978-3-7258-6642-7 (Hbk)
ISBN 978-3-7258-6643-4 (PDF)
https://doi.org/10.3390/books978-3-7258-6643-4

Cover image courtesy of Dominique Singer

Contents

About the Editors

Martin E. G. Blohm

Martin E. G. Blohm (*1966) is Head of the Department of Neonatology and Paediatric Intensive Care Medicine at the Altona Children's Hospital and its associated sites in Hamburg, Germany (since 2024). From 2009 to 2024, he served as senior physician in the Division of Neonatology and Pediatric Critical Care Medicine at the University Medical Center Hamburg-Eppendorf, Germany. His postgraduate qualifications include pediatrics, neonatology, pediatric intensive care, and pediatric cardiology. His scientific work focuses on non-invasive cardiovascular monitoring in neonates and children and on cardiac biomarkers in the perinatal context.

Dominique Singer

Dominique Singer (*1959) is a physiologist and pediatrician. His early career included training at the Department of Vegetative Physiology and Pathophysiology, the Collaborative Research Centre "Organ Protection", and the Department of Pediatrics at University of Göttingen, Germany. He then served as a senior consultant at the Perinatal Center of Würzburg University Children's Hospital from 1999 to 2006. From 2007 to 2025, he held the position of Head of the Division of Neonatology and Pediatric Critical Care Medicine at the University Medical Center Hamburg-Eppendorf (UKE). His scientific interests encompass the comparative physiology of neonatal hypoxia tolerance, the pathophysiology of pediatric hypothermia, and the long-term outcomes of adults born preterm.

Preface

Clinicians and researchers in pediatric intensive care often struggle to find suitable platforms to publish their observations and findings: Adult critical care deems the patients too young and the conditions too rare, neonatology considers the patients too old and the interventions too invasive, and general pediatrics views the courses as too acute and the approach as too technical. To address this issue, we encouraged our colleagues to submit their work to a Special Issue of the journal *Children*. This Reprint presents the resulting collection of papers, covering the full spectrum of the field and documenting its current state. A Spanish resuscitation study confirms the superior efficacy of the two-thumb technique for chest compressions, in line with the latest international guidelines. Three, mostly case-based, papers from Italy, Poland, and Germany focus on infections caused by Group A Streptococci and Respiratory Syncytial Virus. Another study examines the impact of the COVID-19 lockdown on admissions to Pediatric Intensive Care Units (PICUs) in Germany. In this context, the topic of suicidality is also addressed, which a Greek paper analyzes in more detail. The use of organ replacement therapy is outlined in a German cohort of patients with Congenital Diaphragmatic Hernia, suggesting that both early and late need for ECMO is linked to a severe course. Meanwhile, a study of neonates and infants with severe pulmonary hypertension from New York identifies inhaled iloprost as a safe and effective alternative with a potential to avoid the need for ECMO. Finally, the Spanish KIDS TRIAL protocol focuses on arterial hypertension resulting from sleep-disordered breathing, and a US follow-up project addresses the vital issue of PICU survivorship. Although this volume provides only a brief, non-systematic overview of clinical observations and study results, it clearly asserts that pediatric intensive care medicine has become an independent specialty with its own expertise and raison d'être, alongside general pediatrics, neonatology, and adult critical care.

Martin E. G. Blohm and Dominique Singer

Guest Editors

children

MDPI

Article

A Comparison between Three Different Techniques Considering Quality Skills, Fatigue and Hand Pain during a Prolonged Infant Resuscitation: A Cross-Over Study with Lifeguards

Roberto Barcala-Furelos [1], Martín Barcala-Furelos [2,3,*], Francisco Cano-Noguera [4], Martín Otero-Agra [1], Alejandra Alonso-Calvete [1,5], Santiago Martínez-Isasi [6], Silvia Aranda-García [7], Sergio López-García [3] and Antonio Rodríguez-Núñez [8]

1 REMOSS Research Group, Faculty of Education and Sport Sciences, Universidade de Vigo, 36005 Pontevedra, Spain; roberto.barcala.furelos@uvigo.es (R.B.-F.); martinoteroagra@gmail.com (M.O.-A.); alejalonso@uvigo.es (A.A.-C.)
2 Faculty of Health Sciences, Universidad Europea del Atlántico, 39011 Santander, Spain
3 Faculty of Education, Pontifical University of Salamanca, 37002 Salamanca, Spain; slopezga@upsa.es
4 INGESPORT Research Group, Department of Physical Activity and Sports, University of Murcia, 30720 San Javier, Spain; francisco.cano@um.es
5 Facultade de Fisioterapia, Universidade de Vigo, 36005 Pontevedra, Spain
6 Research, Health and Podiatry Unit, Department of Health Sciences, Faculty of Nursing and Podiatry, Universidade da Coruña, 15071 A Coruña, Spain; smtzisasi@gmail.com
7 National Institute of Physical Education of Catalonia, Barcelona University, 08038 Barcelona, Spain; silvia.aranda.garcia@gmail.com
8 Paediatric Intensive Care, Paediatric Intermediate Care and Palliative Care Units, Department of Paediatrics, Hospital Clínico Universitario de Santiago de Compostela, 15706 Santiago de Compostela, Spain; antonio.rodriguez.nunez@sergas.es
* Correspondence: martin.barcala@uneatlantico.es

Abstract: The aim of the study was to compare the quality of CPR (Q-CPR), as well as the perceived fatigue and hand pain in a prolonged infant cardiopulmonary resuscitation (CPR) performed by lifeguards using three different techniques. A randomized crossover simulation study was used to compare three infant CPR techniques: the two-finger technique (TF); the two-thumb encircling technique (TTE) and the two-thumb-fist technique (TTF). 58 professional lifeguards performed three tests in pairs during a 20-min period of CPR. The rescuers performed compressions and ventilations in 15:2 cycles and changed their roles every 2 min. The variables of analysis were CPR quality components, rate of perceived exertion (RPE) and hand pain with numeric rating scale (NRS). All three techniques showed high Q-CPR results (TF: 86 ± 9%/TTE: 88 ± 9%/TTF: 86 ± 16%), and the TTE showed higher values than the TF (p = 0.03). In the RPE analysis, fatigue was not excessive with any of the three techniques (values 20 min between 3.2 for TF, 2.4 in TTE and 2.5 in TTF on a 10-point scale). TF reached a higher value in RPE than TTF in all the intervals analyzed ($p < 0.05$). In relation to NRS, TF showed significantly higher values than TTE and TTF (NRS minute 20 = TF 4.7 vs. TTE 2.5 & TTF 2.2; $p < 0.001$). In conclusion, all techniques have been shown to be effective in high-quality infant CPR in a prolonged resuscitation carried out by lifeguards. However, the two-finger technique is less efficient in relation to fatigue and hand pain compared with two-thumb technique (TF vs. TTF, p = 0.01).

Keywords: lifeguards; infants; resuscitation; chest compression; two fingers; two thumbs

1. Introduction

Pediatric out-of-hospital cardiac arrest (OHCR) is a rare event [1], but when infant OHCR does occur, drowning is a common cause and is a global public health problem drowning and is a global public health problem [2–4] that especially affects toddlers and children aged 0–4 years [5]. Lifeguards usually represent the first line of prevention and intervention in aquatic environments [6,7] and one of their fundamental competencies is cardiopulmonary resuscitation (CPR) [7–10]. Despite this, only the studies by Weber and Moran focused on pediatric CPR applied by lifeguards [11].

In drowning cardiac arrest, systemic hypoxia is the primary factor [12,13], so conventional CPR including ventilations and compressions is the main recommended strategy [13]. The aim of ventilation is to combat hypoxia [14], and the role of compression is to achieve the necessary cerebral and coronary perfusion [15,16].

For the resuscitation of infants, the pediatric section of the European Resuscitation Guidelines 2021 (ERCG2021) [17] recommends the use of the standard two-finger technique (TF) for one rescuer and the two-thumbs encircling technique (TTE) for two rescuers, although it does open the possibility of other techniques as an alternative to traditional methods when resuscitation conditions or fatigue are limiting factors [17]. Ladny et al. have recently proposed a modification of the TTE technique which they have termed "two-thumb-fist" (TTF) [16], which consists of placing the thumbs together and perpendicular at a 90° angle [18] over the lower third of the infant's thorax, and applying force with the weight of the body. All these recommendations for pediatric CPR are focused on the most common OHCA situations, either assisted by bystanders or medical teams. However, to our knowledge there is still a lack of evidence related to which techniques can optimize the quality of pediatric CPR with less fatigue and minimizing the injurious consequences for the rescuer, especially in particular resuscitation situations (e.g., drowning and isolated locations). Our study arises from the belief that current infant CPR techniques can be improved [16] and therefore should be studied and analyzed for each context according to the location where the cardiac arrest occurs (e.g., aquatic environments), the type of rescuer (lifeguards) and the resuscitation time (i.e., prolonged).

The objective of this study is to compare three pediatric resuscitation techniques in a lifeguard-assisted out-of-hospital aquatic setting over a prolonged period of time, to determine the quality of resuscitation as well as the perceived fatigue and hand pain of the rescuers.

2. Materials and Methods

2.1. Study Design

A randomized crossover manikin study was performed to compare the recommended pediatric CPR techniques [17]: two-finger (TF) and two-thumb encircling (TTE) and the new 2-thumb-fist technique (TTF) (Figure 1).

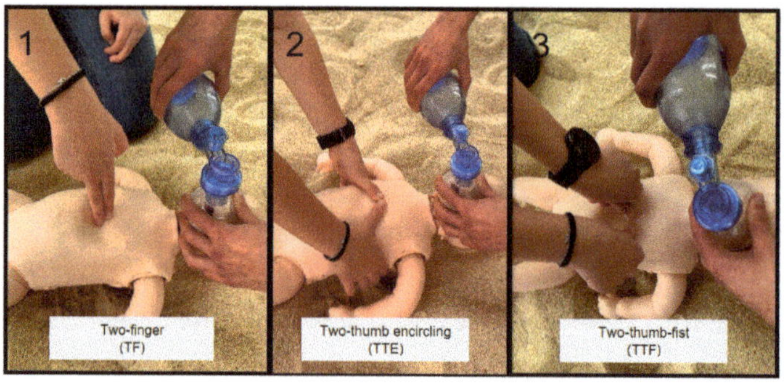

Figure 1. (**1**) Two-finger technique, (**2**) two-thumb encircling, (**3**) two-thumb-fist.

2.2. Participants

This study involved a sample of 58 professional lifeguards from 3 Spanish cities (Pontevedra, Santander and Murcia). 40% (n = 23) were female and 60% (n = 35) were male.

The sample size was based on an assumed minimum of effect size (ES) of 0.25, and error probability of 0.05, and a statistical power of 0.80. These assumptions provided a sample size of 28 study participants computed by G*Power 3.1.9.2 software (Heinrich-Heine-Universität, Düsseldorf, Germany). The final sample was 58 participants, giving a statistical power of 0.99 assuming the effect size and error probability parameters described above. Their mean age was 27 ± 10 years old, their weight was 70 ± 12 kg and their height was 172 ± 9 cm. All participants were informed about the study and gave their written informed consent. The research respected the Helsinki Declaration and the study protocol was approved by the Ethics Committee of the University School of Education and Sport Sciences of the University of Vigo, number 03–0121, date: 18 January 2021.

2.3. Study Protocol

The details can be seen in Figure 2.

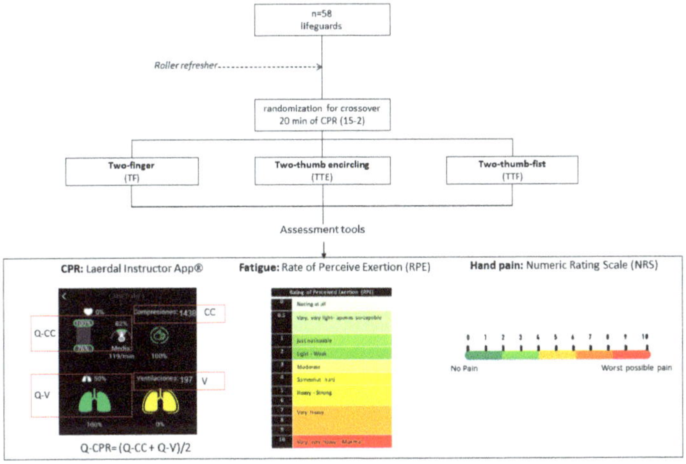

Figure 2. Flow chart design and assessment tools.

2.3.1. Step 1 Roller Refresher

Prior to the study, the rescuers received a one-hour training refresher course given by three instructors who are experts in pediatric CPR. All participants were familiarized with the three techniques, with their partner in the resuscitation team and with the manikin on which the tests would be performed.

2.3.2. Step 2 CPR Trial

Each team of rescuers (pair of lifeguards) performed 3 resuscitation tests of 20 min on an infant manikin. The order of the three tests was randomized. To avoid the effect of fatigue, each test was performed 24 h apart. Each team of rescuers (2 lifeguards) followed the sequence as recommended by ERCG2021 [17] for trained responders: After the first 5 rescue breaths, the team followed the sequence of 15 chest compressions (CC) and 2 ventilations (V). One lifeguard performed CC with the randomized technique while the other rescuer delivered V with an infant-size bag-valve-mask (Laerdal. Stavanger, Norway). Every 8 cycles (approximately 2 min) the roles were exchanged between rescuers. The total test time was 20 min.

2.4. Variables

2.4.1. Cardiopulmonary Resuscitation Variables

Quality parameters were evaluated and disaggregated into Quality of CC (Q-CC), Quality of V (Q-V) and overall CPR Quality (Q-CPR). Each variable was expressed as a percentage and its calculation is based on the following formulas published in previous studies [19]: Q-CPR = [(Q-CC + Q-V) ÷ 2], Q-CC, calculated using the formula; Q-CC = [%CC with adequate depth + %CC with correct chest recoil + %CC with adequate rate (100–120 CC per minute) ÷ 3] and Q-V = V-C ÷ Number of V × 100. Quantitatively, the number of CC and number of V performed during each test were also recorded.

For data analysis, a Laerdal Little Baby QCPR (Stavanger, Norway) manikin () was used, with the Laerdal Instructor App (Stavanger, Norway) configured according to the ERCG2021 [17]. This model corresponds to a baby of 3 months and approximately 5.5 kg.

2.4.2. Rate of Perceived Exertion (RPE) Parameters

At the perceptual level, the modified rating of perceived effort (RPE) [20] was recorded (measurement of the range 0/10—rest/maximal). Previously, the lifeguards were trained in the knowledge and use of this scale. The RPE was measured individually at five different time points: minute 0, 5, 10, 15 and 20 min into the test.

2.4.3. Hand Pain during CPR

Hand pain was measured using a Numeric rating scale (NRS) whose values range from 0 (no pain) to 10 (worst possible pain) [21,22]. NRS is a scale that is easy to interpret, is intuitive and meets the reliability requirements for pain assessment [22]. The hand pain was also measured individually at five different time points: minute 0, 5, 10, 15 and 20 into the test.

2.5. *Statistical Analysis*

Statistical analysis was performed with IBM SPSS Statistics v.20 for Windows (Armonk, NY, USA). To describe the categorical variable (sex), absolute and relative frequencies were used. To describe the continuous variables of the study, measures of central tendency (mean), dispersion (standard deviation) and confidence estimators (95% confidence intervals) were used. The normality of the distributions was tested using the Kolmogorov-Smirnov and Shapiro-Wilk tests as appropriate and, depending on the results of these analyses, parametric or nonparametric tests were performed. In the parametric analyses, the ANOVA repeated measures test was used and in the nonparametric analyses the Friedman repeated measures test with Bonferroni correction in pairs comparisons was used. For significant comparisons, the effect size (ES) was also calculated with the Rosenthal test. For the interpretation of ES, Cohen's recommendations were followed: (<0.2: trivial; 0.2–0.5: small; 0.5–0.8: medium; 0.8–1.3: large; >1.3: very large) A significance level of 0.05 was assigned.

3. Results

The results are based on an analysis of 87 tests, comprising 1740 min of CPR. All the overall results can be seen in Figure 3.

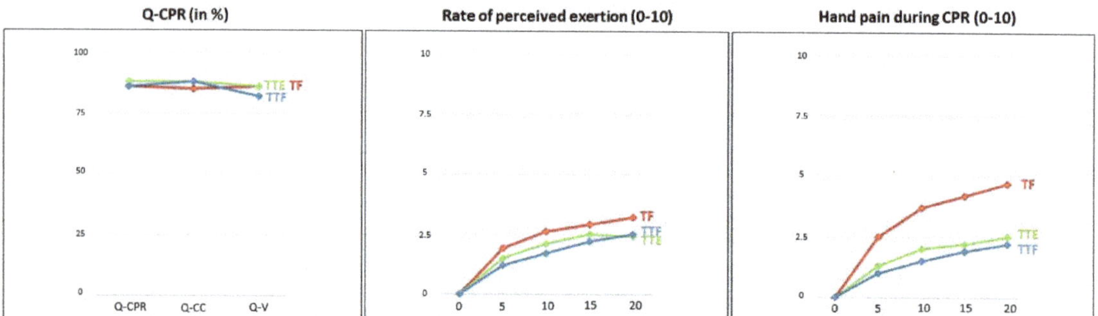

Figure 3. Chart of the results.

3.1. Cardiopulmonary Resuscitation Variables

The results of the CPR tests are shown in Table 1. All techniques obtained high Q-CPR values (TF: 86 ± 9%, TTE: 88 ± 9%/TTF: 86 ± 16%). TTE was statistically superior to TF (TTE vs. TF; $p = 0.03$) although the 2% improvement is not of particular clinical relevance. No differences were found between the techniques in the quality of chest compressions or in the quality of ventilations, with values above 80% in all cases. The quantitative variables of number of CC and number of V were similar, without any statistical significance.

Table 1. Results of CPR test ($n = 29$ pairs).

Variables	TF		TTE		TTF		Friedman or ANOVA Test ($p = 0.05$) (In Brackets) Effect Size with Rosenthal Test
	Mean (SD)	CI (95%)	Mean (SD)	CI (95%)	Mean (SD)	CI (95%)	
Q-CPR (%)	86 (9)	[82–89]	88 (9)	[84–91]	86 (16)	[80–92]	TF vs. TTE = 0.03 (ES 0.23)
Q-CC (%)	85 (11)	[81–89]	88 (9)	[84–91]	88 (9)	[85–92]	NS
Q-V (%)	86 (12)	[76–90]	86 (13)	[82–91]	82 (23)	[73–91]	NS
CC	1438 (155)	[1379–1496]	1437 (104)	[1398–1477]	1442 (131)	[1392–1491]	NS
V	197 (21)	[189–205]	197 (14)	[191–202]	197 (17)	[191–204]	NS

TF: two-finger, TTE: two-thumb, TTF: two-thumb-fist Q-CC: Quality of chest compressions; Q-CPR: CPR global quality; Q-V: Quality of ventilations; CC: Number of chest compression; V: Number of ventilations. SD: Standard deviation, CI: 95% Confidence intervals, NS: Not significance.

3.2. Rate of Perceived Exertion (RPE)

The RPE results are shown in Table 2 and Figure 3. In the intragroup analysis, the significant increase in RPE occurs progressively in all techniques at each control point, compared with baseline state (minute 0). No statistical significance was found in any technique in the intragroup comparison between minutes 15 and 20 ($p > 0.05$). In the comparison of the techniques (intergroup) in each of the sections, statistically significant differences were found between TF and TTF. The TF technique generated a higher RPE from min 5 to min 20 (min 5 $p = 0.003$, min 10 $p < 0.001$, min 15 $p = 0.02$, min 20 $p = 0.01$).

Table 2. Results of Rating of Perceive Exertion (RPE). ($n = 56$; 2 missed).

Variables	TF		TTE		TTF		Friedman Test with Bonferroni Correction ($p = 0.05$)
	Mean (SD)	CI (95%)	Mean (SD)	CI (95%)	Mean (SD)	CI (95%)	
RPE minute 0	0.0 (0.1)	[0.0–0.1]	0.1 (0.3)	[0.0–0.2]	0.0 (0.2)	[0.0–0.1]	NS
RPE minute 5	1.9 (1.6)	[1.5–2.3]	1.5 (1.2)	[1.2–1.8]	1.2 (1.2)	[0.9–1.5]	TF vs. TTF = 0.003 (0.46)
RPE minute 10	2.6 (1.7)	[2.2–3.1]	2.1 (1.3)	[1.8–2.5]	1.7 (1.4)	[1.3–2.1]	TF vs. TTF < 0.001 (0.53)
RPE minute 15	2.9 (1.7)	[2.5–3.4]	2.5 (1.6)	[2.0–2.9]	2.2 (1.6)	[1.8–2.6]	TF vs. TTF = 0.02 (0.37)
RPE minute 20	3.2 (1.8)	[2.7–3.7]	2.4 (1.7)	[2.0–2.9]	2.5 (1.7)	[2.0–2.9]	TF vs. TTF = 0.01 (0.38)
Friedman Test with Bonferroni correction ($p = 0.05$)	0 vs. (5,10,15,20) < 0.001 5 vs. 10 = 0.03 5 vs. (15,20) < 0.001		0 vs. (5,10,15,20) < 0.001 5 vs. (15,20) < 0.001		0 vs. (5,10,15,20) ≤ 0.001 5 vs. (15,20) < 0.001 10 vs. 20 = 0.002		

TF: two-finger, TTE: two-thumb, TTF: two-thumb-fist. RPE: Rating of perceive exertion SD: Standard deviation, CI: 95% Confidence intervals, NS: Not significance.

3.3. Numeric Rating Scale (NRS) for Hand Pain

The results of hand pain are shown in Table 3 and Figure 3.

In the intragroup analysis, the significant increase in NRS occurred in all three techniques analyzed at each control point ($p < 0.05$); in the comparison of the techniques (intergroup) significantly higher values of hand pain were observed throughout the test when using TF compared to TTE (min 0 vs. 5: $p = 0.007$, min 5 vs. 10: < 0.001, min 10 vs. 15: $p < 0.001$ and min 15 vs. 20: $p < 0.001$) and with TTF ($p < 0.001$ for all intervals). The ES value was medium (0.5 to <0.8) in the comparison of TF with TTE while from min 5 onwards it was large (0.8 to <1.3) in the TF and TTF comparison.

Table 3. Results of Numeric rating scale (NRS). (n = 56; 2 missed).

Variables	TF		TTE		TTF		Friedman Test with Bonferroni Correction (p = 0.05)
	Mean (SD)	CI (95%)	Mean (SD)	CI (95%)	Mean (SD)	Mean (SD)	
NRS minute 0	0.0 (0.2)	[0.0–0.1]	0.1 (0.1)	[0.0–0.1]	0.0 (0.1)	[0.0–0.1]	NS
NRS minute 5	2.5 (1.8)	[2.0–3.0]	1.3 (1.1)	[1.0–1.6]	1.0 (1.1)	[0.7–1.3]	TF vs. TTE = 0.007 (0.44) TF vs. TTF < 0.001 (0.73)
NRS minute 10	3.7 (2.2)	[3.1–4.2]	2.0 (1.3)	[1.6–2.3]	1.5 (1.4)	[1.1–1.9]	TF vs. TTE < 0.001 (0.63) TF vs. TTF < 0.001 (0.91)
NRS minute 15	4.2 (2.2)	[3.6–4.8]	2.2 (1.3)	[1.8–2.5]	1.9 (1.4)	[1.5–2.2]	TF vs. TTE < 0.001 (0.70) TF vs. TTF < 0.001 (0.90)
NRS minute 20	4.7 (2.5)	[4.0–5.4]	2.5 (1.5)	[2.1–2.9]	2.2 (1.5)	[1.7–2.6]	TF vs. TTE < 0.001 (0.69) TF vs. TTF < 0.001 (0.80)
Friedman Test with Bonferroni correction (p = 0.05)	0 vs. (5,10,15,20) ≤ 0.001 5 vs. 10 = 0.013 5 vs. (15,20) < 0.001 10 vs. 20 < 0.001		0 vs. (5,10,15,20) < 0.001 5 vs. 10 = 0.021 5 vs. (15,20) < 0.001 10 vs. 20 = 0.041		0 vs. (5,10,15,20) ≤ 0.001 5 vs. (15,20) < 0.001 10 vs. 20 = 0.003		

TF: two-finger, TTE: two-thumb, TTF: two-thumb-fist, NRS: Numeric rating scale, SD: Standard deviation, CI: 95% Confidence intervals, NS: Not significance.

4. Discussion

This study was to assess the quality of resuscitation, the perceived fatigue and the hand pain with three pediatric CPR techniques in an aquatic environment assisted by lifeguards. The main findings were: (a) the rescuers are able to maintain a high quality of CPR regardless of the technique employed, (b) perceived fatigue is low in all three techniques, although slightly higher in TF and (c) hand pain using the TF technique is moderate compared to TTE and TTF which was mild.

Survival from pediatric cardiac arrest and a favorable neurological outcome is associated with the duration of CPR [23], as well as witnessed cardiac arrest Delivery of high quality CPR is likely to be another major factor [24]. Therefore, the analysis of the different methods of providing CC in infants has two important challenges; the first one achieving and maintaining high quality CPR without developing fatigue.

Traditionally the TF technique has been recommended when there is only one rescuer [17] and one of the main reasons is to minimize the no-flow time [25], although the time saved compared to TTE is just over half a second [26] and it could be further reduced if two rescuers are carrying out the resuscitation. On the other hand, TTE is recommended when CPR is performed by at least two trained first responders [17], although some studies consider it superior even if performed individually [26–28]. One of the main strengths of TTE is the improvement in the depth of CC [26–31] compared to TF. This is something that the new TTF method developed by Ladny et al. and Smereka et al. has also achieved [16,18], with the placement of the thumbs at 90°. However there is no superiority in either quality or depth between the methods using the two thumbs TTE or the TTF [32,33]. In our study, we analyzed the Q-CPR in a comprehensive manner. All three techniques achieved values above 85% with no statistically significant differences between groups. The quantification of good CPR in a simulation with manikins has been arbitrarily assumed to be equal to or higher than a value of 70% [34]. One possible explanation is that rescuers have comprehensive training which includes endurance and strength capabilities [35], and their work also specifically requires training in both the lower and upper limbs (including hand muscles), in addition to good physical health to allow CPR to be performed [36] even to allow CPR to be performed under conditions of previous fatigue [8].

One of the analysis points was to find out the intensity of the fatigue and if there were any differences in the technique used. Our findings showed low intensity fatigue (between light and moderate) with no differences between the ways of providing CC. The study by Reynols et al. [37] also found no differences between the techniques analyzed (TT vs. TTE) during 5-min of CPR, but did assume a higher intensity of "hard" fatigue for TT and "somewhat hard" i.e., hard for TTE. Jung et al. did find high fatigue values during a 5-min test with a single-rescuer, especially in the TF technique [38]. Possibly the most relevant difference is the time during which CC is performed without without changing rescuers and it seems that fatigue is also related to the type of victim and increases with greater size [37].

Santos-Folgar et al. analyzed the anatomical area of the upper limb with the greatest fatigue to during 10-min of CPR with the TF technique and found that the only point where fatigue was high was the area between the fingers and the palm of the hand (8 points out of 10) [39]. The Santos-Folgar's study used the Visual Analogue Scale (VAS) as a fatigue assessment tool. The most common use of this scale is the assessment of pain and the population studied was nursing students, which could perhaps be a confounding bias with fatigue. For this reason, pain was included as a variable using the NRS as a tool because of its better sensitivity [21] in addition to being one of the most widely used scales [40]. As expected, TF resulted in significantly higher pain, which at the end of the test was an increase of 25% compared to the other two techniques. These results are in agreement with previous studies that found the hand to be the least comfortable place during TF [28,38]. The use of the body weight on the fingers in TTF or the pressure of the two hands encircling the infant's thorax using the anatomical gripper with the thumbs in TTE seems more efficient. Moreover, there is greater involvement of larger muscles or powerful kinetic chains compared to TF whose compression force is lower [29] since it is projected exclusively from the wrist to the two fingers as well as in a smaller contact area [38].

Indeed one of the practical implications of this study is to understand the effects of prolonged pediatric CPR and to optimize it in order to offer the most comfortable alternatives to rescuers, who often operate in remote locations with scarce resources. "Pain cannot be treated if it cannot be assessed" [22] and applied to this study, TTE or TTF would be the preferred choice. The current results should encourage lifeguard organizations to explore these different techniques within their protocols and incorporate fatigue and pain assessment scales to promote best professional practice in the safest, most efficient manner and to avoid injuries that may detract from lifeguard service.

Limitations of the Study

This study has limitations that should be pointed out. First, it is a simulation study with physically fit rescuers in a controlled context; therefore, in a real situation, with a different first responder profile and in a different resuscitation environment, the results may be different. In this study, not all variables which determine the quality of CPR were collected by an APP software limitation, especially the depth of compression in millimeters, so results must be construed with this important restriction. Another limitation for understand the results was the manikin represents a three-month-old baby. This study should be tested with older and larger toddlers. The limited sample of this study is another important limitation, so further research is needed in order to validate the results obtained. The strength of this study is the novelty and relevance of the topic, as well as the limited evidence in this context. Simulation-based analysis with manikins is useful when the possibility of analysis in situations with real patients has not existed so far.

5. Conclusions

All techniques have been shown to be effective in high-quality infant CPR during a prolonged resuscitation provided by lifeguards. However, the two-finger technique is less efficient in relation to rescuers comfort with high fatigue and hand pain compared to two-thumb techniques (TTE and TTF). This study supports the recommendation that the traditional two-finger technique in the context of prolonged resuscitations should not be the preferred option when there is more than one rescuer.

Author Contributions: Conceptualization, R.B.-F., M.B.-F., M.O.-A., A.A.-C., S.M.-I., S.A.-G., S.L.-G. and A.R.-N.; Data curation, F.C.-N. and A.R.-N.; Formal analysis, R.B.-F., M.O.-A., A.A.-C. and S.M.-I.; Investigation, M.B.-F., A.A.-C., S.M.-I., S.A.-G. and S.L.-G.; Methodology, R.B.-F. and M.O.-A.;

Resources, M.B.-F. and F.C.-N.; Supervision, S.A.-G.; Validation, M.O.-A.; Writing—original draft, R.B.-F. All authors have read and agreed to the published version of the manuscript.

Funding: This research received no external funding.

Institutional Review Board Statement: The study was conducted in accordance with the Declaration of Helsinki and approved by the Ethics Committee of the University School of Education and Sport Sciences of the University of Vigo (number 03-0121, date: 18 January 2021).

Informed Consent Statement: Informed consent was obtained from all subjects involved in the study.

Data Availability Statement: Not applicable.

Conflicts of Interest: The authors declare no conflict of interest.

References

1. Lee, J.; Yang, W.-C.; Lee, E.-P.; Huang, J.-L.; Hsiao, H.-J.; Lin, M.-J.; Wu, H.-P. Clinical survey and predictors of outcomes of pediatric out-of-hospital cardiac arrest admitted to the emergency department. *Sci. Rep.* **2019**, *9*, 7032. [CrossRef] [PubMed]
2. World Health Organization. *Preventing Drowning: An Implementation Guide*; World Health Organization: Geneva, Switzerland, 2017; p. 105.
3. Wu, Y.; Huang, Y.; Schwebel, D.C.; Hu, G. Unintentional child and adolescent drowning mortality from 2000 to 2013 in 21 countries: Analysis of the WHO mortality database. *Int. J. Environ. Res. Public Health* **2017**, *14*, 875. [CrossRef] [PubMed]
4. Global Report on Drowning: Preventing a Leading Killer. Australian Policy Online 2014. Available online: https://doi.org/10.3390/ijerph140808755 (accessed on 6 December 2014).
5. UNICEF; World Health Organization. *World Report on Child Injury Prevention*; Peden, M.M., Oyegbite, K., Ozanne-Smith, J., Hyder, A.A., Branche, C., Rahman, A.K.M.F., Rivara, F., Bartolomeos, K., Eds.; World Health Organization: Geneva, Switzerland, 2008; 211p.
6. Barcala-Furelos, R.; Aranda-García, S.; Abelairas-Gómez, C.; Martínez-Isasi, S.; López-Mesa, F.; Oleagordia-Aguirre, A.; Palacios-Aguilar, J.; Szpilman, D. Occupational health recommendations for lifeguards in aquatic emergencies in the Covid-19 era: Prevention, rescue and resuscitation. *Revista Espanola Salud Publica* **2020**, *94*, e202006074.
7. Li, S.; Kan, T.; Guo, Z.; Chen, C.; Gui, L. Assessing the quality of CPR performed by a single lifeguard, two lifeguards and a lifeguard with a bystander after water rescue: A quasi-experimental trial. *Emerg. Med. J.* **2020**, *37*, 306–313. [CrossRef]
8. Barcala-Furelos, R.; Szpilman, D.; Palacios-Aguilar, J.; Costas-Veiga, J.; Gómez, C.A.; Bores-Cerezal, A.; López-García, S.; Rodriguez-Nunez, A. Assessing the efficacy of rescue equipment in lifeguard resuscitation efforts for drowning. *Am. J. Emerg. Med.* **2015**, *34*, 480–485. [CrossRef]
9. Szpilman, D.; Tipton, M.; Sempsrott, J.; Webber, J.; Bierens, J.; Dawes, P.; Seabra, R.; Barcala-Furelos, R.; Queiroga, A.C. Drowning timeline: A new systematic model of the drowning process. *Am. J. Emerg. Med.* **2016**, *34*, 2224–2226. [CrossRef]
10. Faddy, S.C. Towards new models of cardiopulmonary resuscitation teaching: The role of practical scenario training on surf lifesavers' perceptions of resuscitation efficacy. *Resuscitation* **2002**, *53*, 159–165. [CrossRef]
11. Webber, J.; Moran, K.; Cumin, D. Paediatric cardiopulmonary resuscitation: Knowledge and perceptions of surf lifeguards. *J. Paediatr. Child Health* **2018**, *55*, 156–161. [CrossRef]
12. Szpilman, D.; Bierens, J.J.; Handley, A.J.; Orlowski, J.P. Drowning. *N. Engl. J. Med.* **2012**, *366*, 2102–2110. [CrossRef]
13. Bierens, J.; Abelairas-Gomez, C.; Furelos, R.B.; Beerman, S.; Claesson, A.; Dunne, C.; Elsenga, H.; Morgan, P.; Mecrow, T.; Pereira, J.; et al. Resuscitation and emergency care in drowning: A scoping review. *Resuscitation* **2021**, *162*, 205–217. [CrossRef]
14. Szpilman, D.; Soares, M. In-water resuscitation—Is it worthwhile? *Resuscitation* **2004**, *63*, 25–31. [CrossRef] [PubMed]
15. Saini, S.S.; Gupta, N.; Kumar, P.; Bhalla, A.K.; Kaur, H. A comparison of two-fingers technique and two-thumbs encircling hands technique of chest compression in neonates. *J. Perinatol.* **2011**, *32*, 690–694. [CrossRef] [PubMed]
16. Ladny, J.R.; Smereka, J.; Rodríguez-Núñez, A.; Leung, S.; Ruetzler, K.; Szarpak, L. Is there any alternative to standard chest compression techniques in infants? A randomized manikin trial of the new "2-thumb-fist" option. *Medicine* **2018**, *97*, e9386. [CrossRef] [PubMed]
17. Van de Voorde, P.; Turner, N.M.; Djakow, J.; de Lucas, N.; Martinez-Mejias, A.; Biarent, D.; Bingham, R.; Brissaud, O.; Hoffmann, F.; Johannesdottir, G.B.; et al. European resuscitation council guidelines 2021: Paediatric life support. *Resuscitation* **2021**, *161*, 327–387. [CrossRef]
18. Smereka, J.; Szarpak, L.; Smereka, A.; Leung, S.; Ruetzler, K. Evaluation of new two-thumb chest compression technique for infant CPR performed by novice physicians. A randomized, crossover, manikin trial. *Am. J. Emerg. Med.* **2017**, *35*, 604–609. [CrossRef]
19. Barcala-Furelos, R.; Abelairas-Gomez, C.; Aranda-García, S.; Lorenzo-Martínez, M.; Martinez-Isasi, S.; Durán-Álvarez, C.; Palacios-Aguilar, J.; Rodríguez-Núñez, A. Is it feasible "scoop and run while playing" resuscitation on a rescue water craft? A randomized simulation study with lifeguards. *Am. J. Emerg. Med.* **2020**, *38*, 618–623. [CrossRef]
20. Foster, C.; Florhaug, J.A.; Franklin, J.; Gottschall, L.; Hrovatin, L.A.; Parker, S.; Doleshal, P.; Dodge, C. A new approach to monitoring exercise training. *J. Strength Cond. Res.* **2001**, *15*, 109–115.
21. Williamson, A.; Hoggart, B. Pain: A review of three commonly used pain rating scales. *J. Clin. Nurs.* **2005**, *14*, 798–804. [CrossRef]

22. Karcioglu, O.; Topacoglu, H.; Dikme, O.; Dikme, O. A systematic review of the pain scales in adults: Which to use? *Am. J. Emerg. Med.* **2018**, *36*, 707–714. [CrossRef]
23. López-Herce, J.; García, C.; Dominguez-Sampedro, P.; Rodriguez-Nunez, A.; Carrillo, A.; Calvo, C.; Delgado, M.A. Spanish study group of cardiopulmonary arrest in children outcome of out-of-hospital cardiorespiratory arrest in children. *Pediatr. Emerg. Care* **2005**, *21*, 807–815. [CrossRef]
24. Sahu, S.; Kishore, K.; Lata, I. Better outcome after pediatric resuscitation is still a dilemma. *J. Emerg. Trauma Shock* **2010**, *3*, 243–250. [CrossRef] [PubMed]
25. Ruetzler, K.; Smereka, J.; Szarpak, L.; Czekajlo, M. Novel method of infant chest compression. Does the arrangement of the thumbs matter? *Am. J. Emerg. Med.* **2019**, *37*, 769–770. [CrossRef] [PubMed]
26. Udassi, S.; Udassi, J.P.; Lamb, M.A.; Theriaque, D.W.; Shuster, J.J.; Zaritsky, A.L.; Haque, I.U. Two-thumb technique is superior to two-finger technique during lone rescuer infant manikin CPR. *Resuscitation* **2010**, *81*, 712–717. [CrossRef]
27. Lee, J.E.; Lee, J.; Oh, J.; Park, C.H.; Kang, H.; Lim, T.H.; Yoo, K.H. Comparison of two-thumb encircling and two-finger technique during infant cardiopulmonary resuscitation with single rescuer in simulation studies: A systematic review and meta-analysis. *Medicine* **2019**, *98*, e17853. [CrossRef]
28. Pellegrino, J.L.; Bogumil, D.; Epstein, J.L.; Burke, R.V. Two-thumb-encircling advantageous for lay responder infant CPR: A randomised manikin study. *Arch. Dis. Child.* **2018**, *104*, 530–534. [CrossRef] [PubMed]
29. Tsou, J.-Y.; Kao, C.-L.; Chang, C.-J.; Tu, Y.-F.; Su, F.-C.; Chi, C.-H. Biomechanics of two-thumb versus two-finger chest compression for cardiopulmonary resuscitation in an infant manikin model. *Eur. J. Emerg. Med.* **2020**, *27*, 132–136. [CrossRef]
30. Chang, C.-Y.; Lin, P.-C.; Chien, Y.-J.; Chen, C.-S.; Wu, M.-Y. Analysis of chest-compression depth and full recoil in two infant chest-compression techniques performed by a single rescuer: Systematic review and meta-analysis. *Int. J. Environ. Res. Public Health* **2020**, *17*, 4018. [CrossRef]
31. Chang, C.Y.; Hou, Y.T.; Chien, Y.J.; Chen, Y.L.; Lin, P.C.; Chen, C.S.; Wu, M.Y. Two-thumb or two-finger technique in infant cardio-pulmonary resuscitation by a single rescuer? A meta-analysis with GOSH analysis. *Int. J. Environ. Res. Public Health* **2020**, *17*, 5214. [CrossRef]
32. Rodriguez-Ruiz, E.; Martín, V.G.; Abelairas-Gómez, C.; Vidal, F.S.; González, C.G.; Barcala-Furelos, R.; Rodríguez-Nuñez, A. A new chest compression technique in infants. *Med. Intensiv. (Engl. Ed.)* **2019**, *43*, 346–351. [CrossRef]
33. Rodriguez-Ruiz, E.; Martínez-Puga, A.; Carballo-Fazanes, A.; Abelairas-Gómez, C.; Rodríguez-Nuñez, A. Two new chest compression methods might challenge the standard in a simulated infant model. *Eur. J. Pediatr.* **2019**, *178*, 1529–1535. [CrossRef]
34. Perkins, G.D.; Colquhoun, M.; Simons, R. *ABC of Resuscitation*, 5th ed.; BMJ Books: London, UK, 2004; pp. 97–101.
35. Reilly, T.; Wooler, A.; Tipton, M. Occupational fitness standards for beach lifeguards. Phase 1: The physiological demands of beach lifeguarding. *Occup. Med.* **2005**, *56*, 6–11. [CrossRef] [PubMed]
36. López-García, S.; Ruibal-Lista, B.; Palacios-Aguilar, J.; Santiago-Alonso, M.; Prieto, J. Relationship between the performance in a maximum effort test for lifeguards and the time spent in a water rescue. *Int. J. Environ. Res. Public Health* **2021**, *18*, 3407. [CrossRef] [PubMed]
37. Reynolds, C.; Cox, J.; Livingstone, V.; Dempsey, E.M. Rescuer exertion and fatigue using two-thumb vs. two-finger method during simulated neonatal cardiopulmonary resuscitation. *Front. Pediatr.* **2020**, *8*, 133. [CrossRef] [PubMed]
38. Santos-Folgar, M.; Otero-Agra, M.; Prada-Pérez, A.; Barcala-Furelos, R.; Rodríguez-Núñez, A.; Fernández-Méndez, F. Fatigue during infant cardiopulmonary resuscitation: Is it really a problem for quality performance? *Pediatr. Emerg. Care* **2021**, *37*, e278–e279. [CrossRef]
39. Jung, W.J.; Hwang, S.O.; Kim, H.I.; Cha, Y.S.; Kim, O.H.; Kim, H.; Lee, K.H.; Cha, K.-C. 'Knocking-fingers' chest compression technique in infant cardiac arrest: Single-rescuer manikin study. *Eur. J. Emerg. Med.* **2019**, *26*, 261–265. [CrossRef]
40. Hamdan, K.M. Nurses' assessment practices of pain among critically Ill patients. *Pain Manag. Nurs.* **2019**, *20*, 489–496. [CrossRef]

children

MDPI

Systematic Review

State of the Art of Invasive Group A Streptococcus Infection in Children: A Scoping Review of the Literature with a Focus on Predictors of Invasive Infection

Francesco Mariani [1], Carolina Gentili [1], Valentina Pulcinelli [1], Laura Martino [1], Piero Valentini [1] and Danilo Buonsenso [1,2,*]

1 Department of Woman and Child Health and Public Health, Fondazione Policlinico Universitario A. Gemelli IRCCS, 00168 Rome, Italy; francesco.mariani.100292@gmail.com (F.M.); carolina.gentili01@gmail.com (C.G.); valentina.pulcinelli01@icatt.it (V.P.); martino.laura96@gmail.com (L.M.); piero.valentini@unicatt.it (P.V.)

2 Centro di Salute Globale, Università Cattolica del Sacro Cuore, 00168 Rome, Italy

* Correspondence: danilobuonsenso@gmail.com; Tel.: +39-0630-154-390

Abstract: Currently, it remains unclear why some children develop invasive group A Streptococcus (iGAS) and how to manage this condition. Therefore, to explore available works in the literature, we performed a scoping review aiming to analyze the current literature on clinical presentation of different illnesses outcomes of iGAS, with a specific focus on predictors of invasive infection, including an assessment of the prodromal stages of the disease and the possible presence of previous non-invasive GAS infections in children that later developed iGAS. Methods: We conducted a systematic search on PubMed and SCOPUS of all pediatric studies reporting iGAS cases, following the Preferred Reporting Items for Systematic reviews and Meta-Analyses extension for Scoping Reviews (PRISMA-ScR) checklist. For those studies in which multivariable analysis investigating iGAS risk factors was performed, a second review was performed and reported in detail. Results: A total of 209 studies were included. Five studies investigated risk factors for iGAS, the most relevant being varicella infection, chronic underlying illness, presence of the speC gene in GAS strains, acetaminophen and ibuprofen use, children nonwhite, living in low-income households, exposure to varicella at home, persistent high fever, having more than one other child in the home, and new use of NSAIDs. Although we observed a progressive increase in the number of papers published on this topic, no trials investigating the benefits of clindamycin or intravenous immunoglobulins were found and low-to-middle-income countries were found to be poorly represented in the current literature. Conclusions: Our scoping review highlights important gaps regarding several aspects of iGAS in children, including prodromic presentation and optimal treatment strategies. There is also little representation of low–middle-income countries. The current literature does not allow the performance of systematic reviews or meta-analyses, but this work should inform healthcare professionals, policy makers, and funding agencies on which studies to prioritize on this topic.

Keywords: group A Streptococcus; GAS; invasive group A Streptococcus; iGAS; IVIG; clindamycin

1. Introduction

Streptococcus pyogenes (group A Streptococcus, GAS) can cause a broad spectrum of infections, ranging from minor illnesses such as pharyngitis and superficial skin infections to severe and invasive diseases, including pneumonia, meningitis, sepsis, streptococcal toxic shock syndrome, and necrotizing fasciitis [1]. An invasive disease is defined as the isolation of GAS from a normally sterile site of the body and it occurs when bacteria spread throughout the bloodstream, the cerebrospinal fluid, the lungs, and soft tissue [1]. A critical virulence factor is the M protein [2,3]. Invasive group A Streptococcus infection (iGAS) is a life-threatening condition, with high case fatality rates and high morbidity. In fact, invasive disease can lead to several long-term sequelae, being an important cause of premature disability in pediatric populations [1].

Surveillance is essential to establish the real burden of this disease in children. According to the CDC's Active Bacterial Core surveillance reports, overall iGAS incidence increased every year from 2012 to 2019; in 2020, especially during the first months of the pandemic period, the incidence of invasive disease saw a historical drop and the change was greatest for children aged 5 to 17 years [4]. Unexpectedly, the preliminary data from the surveillance reports of 2022 showed a monthly increase in the incidence of iGAS infection in children from September to November, thus leading the CDC to issue a health advisory [5]. Data from the first months of 2023 confirmed a higher incidence of these infections, compared to pre-pandemic levels. Different European countries reported to the ECDC an increase in iGAS disease in children aged less than 10 years from September 2022, with Ireland, France, and the UK reporting several deaths, too [6]. In the Netherlands, in 2022, a more than twofold increase in the number of iGAS infections compared to pre-pandemic reports was observed, with a higher increase in children under 5 years of age [7]. Otherwise, the UK experienced a surge in the number of invasive infections in children younger than 15 years [8]. However, the ongoing investigations have not yet found a new strain or increased antibiotic resistance, so the WHO has assessed the risk for the general population posed by iGAS infections as low [9]. Nevertheless, the report of higher than usual numbers of cases of iGAS has alarmed both the public and clinicians, with consequences for routine care. Higher rates of antibiotic prescriptions have been reported [10]. As a possible consequence, during these months of iGAS case number surges, a shortage of amoxicillin has been reported in most European countries [10].

One of the reasons that may have induced such public opinion is parents' fear of GAS infection, and theoretical attempts for early diagnosis and treatment are goals of preventing non-invasive GAS infection from evolving into iGAS. However, so far, little is known about the natural history of iGAS and whether an invasive infection is the consequence of a non-recognized GAS infection or colonization. So far, we know that an increase in the incidence of iGAS is related to the high circulation of respiratory viruses, especially Respiratory Syncytial Virus (RSV) and seasonal influenza [11,12] and chickenpox can be a facilitating factor for the development of iGAS. Conversely, what is less known is whether it is possible to prevent the development of iGAS by early recognition and treatment of GAS infection. This last observation has direct implication on routine care because if iGAS suddenly begins as a sudden invasive infection without a previous phase of non-invasive GAS infection/colonization, there is no need for the public and healthcare professionals to be exaggeratedly scared of iGAS and, therefore, antibiotic use may be reduced. Conversely, if the literature suggests that iGAS develops after a non-treated possible or certain GAS infection, this suggests that better strategies are needed to achieve the goal of preventing the development of iGAS.

For these reasons, we performed a scoping review aiming to analyze the current literature on clinical presentation of different localizations and the main outcomes of iGAS, with a specific focus on predictors of invasive infection, including an assessment of the prodromic stages of the disease and the possible presence of previous non-invasive GAS infections in children that later developed iGAS. Our team opted for a scoping review because it is currently unknown if there is any evidence that early treatment of non-complicated GAS infections can prevent iGAS or if iGAS is the consequence of an undiagnosed non-complicated GAS infection or if iGAS should be treated with intravenous immunoglobulins (IVIG) and clindamycin (or one of them) or not. Therefore, we decided to explore what types of paper are currently available as well as where and when available studies have been performed, aiming to inform researchers if systematic reviews and meta-analyses on this topic are feasible or not and to inform what studies are needed to fill current gaps.

2. Materials and Methods

2.1. Search Strategy and Selection Criteria for Included Studies

Our review aims to study a very broad topic to provide the scientific community with a picture of the current literature available in this regard. For this reason, a scoping review, conducted in line with a previously published protocol [13] and well-defined guidelines, seemed to us the best methodological choice. For reporting, we decided to follow the indication of the Preferred Reporting Items for Systematic reviews and Meta-Analyses extension for Scoping Reviews (PRISMA-ScR) checklist [14].

A single author (FM) developed a search strategy, subsequently discussed and approved by all the team, based on a combination of the following terms: "pediatric", "iGAS (and its possible clinical manifestations)", and "group A *Streptococcus pyogenes*". We considered children and pediatric patients younger than 18 years. The search strategy for PubMed is available in the extended data section of the protocol. The terms used for this search were adapted for use with other bibliographic databases thanks to the Polyglot Function of Systematic Review Accelerator. PubMed and SCOPUS were the two databases screened and only articles written in English were included. We did not apply any data restrictions and included studies published until 31 January 2023. PubMed and SCOPUS searches were performed on the same day.

The main review question is "which are the predictors of clinical iGAS"?

This review also assess the following sub-questions:

1. Which are the most frequently reported localizations of different types of iGAS?
2. Which outcomes are reported in the literature about the different types of iGAS (pneumonia, meningitis, sepsis, and abscesses)?

This review includes studies performed on children and adolescents (younger than 18 years) with a confirmed diagnosis of iGAS defined as a laboratory isolation of GAS from any normal sterile site or isolation of GAS from a non-sterile site in patients with necrotizing fasciitis or streptococcal toxic shock syndrome. We include children diagnosed with pneumonia, sepsis, abscesses, or meningitis, due to GAS invasion.

One author screened for possible duplicates. Following the indication of the inclusion criteria, two reviewers (CG and VP) independently screened titles and abstracts and subsequently full texts to select works that could be included in the review. In case of a discrepancy between the two (we had 482 conflicts), a third reviewer (DB) decided whether to include the works.

2.2. Data Extraction

An initial data extraction was performed by a single reviewer (CG for half the included papers and VP for the other half) who compiled an initial Excel sheet in which the following information was collected: year of publication, type of study, region of origin, either retrospective or prospective study, either monocentric or multicentric study, if a multivariable analysis was performed or not, number of centers included, sample size, enrollment start and end date, length of participants' follow-up, study eligibility criteria, age of patients, number of female patients, if analysis of comorbidities was performed or not, number of patients with comorbidities, if antibiotics were given, if intravenous immunoglobulins were given, if clindamycin was given, number of patients who died because of the disease, number of patients who died for other reasons, number of patients who survived with sequelae, and what type of sequelae were developed.

Considering the high number of studies included, we decided to perform a second data extraction including only papers in which multivariable analysis investigating iGAS risk factors was performed. For those articles, the following information was collected and presented in a single table: number of patients with invasive infection, inclusion criteria, previous or starting symptoms or conditions which could lead to iGAS, associated factors detected through univariable or multivariable analysis, Streptococcal infection previously detected and not treated, previous therapy, and death from Streptococcal disease or sequelae due to the invasive infection.

A critical appraisal was not pursued due to its limited relevance within the scope of a scoping review, postponing this objective to any future systematic reviews.

3. Results

Two-hundred and nine studies were included in our scoping review (Figure 1) and the general characteristics of the studies included are reported in Table 1. The full list of studies included in the scoping review is available in the Supplementary Materials.

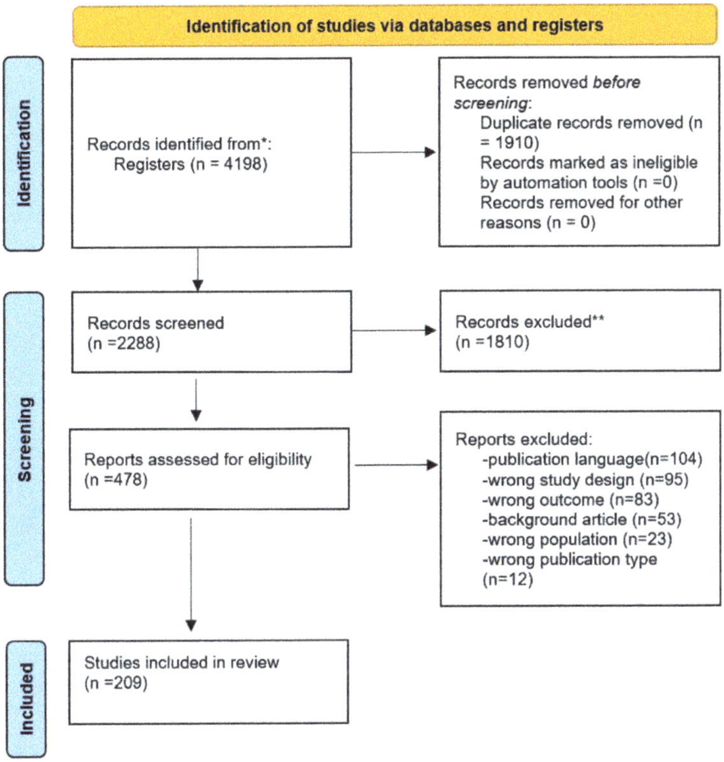

Figure 1. Study flowchart. *, ** not fulfilling study criteria.

Table 1. Study characteristics.

	Number of Studies (N = 209)
Type of study	
RCT	0
NRCT	0
Observational	54
Case report	141
Case series	14
Study design	
Retrospective	205
Prospective	4

Table 1. *Cont.*

	Number of Studies (N = 209)
Number of centers	
Monocentric	177
Multicentric	32
Region	
Europe	60
Africa	6
North America	87
Central or South America	2
Asia	47
Oceania	7
Multivariable analysis for iGAS risk factors performed	5
Information about comorbidities collected	115

Included papers described iGAS cases characterized by the following clinical localizations: CNS localizations (thirty-six studies), streptococcal toxic shock syndrome (thirty-five studies), skin (twenty-five studies), sepsis (twenty-three studies), cardiac (eight studies), gastrointestinal (six studies), pneumonia (six studies), osteomyelitis (five studies), kidneys (one study), and a variety of clinical iGAS localizations in fifty-five studies.

It is possible to observe a progressive incrementation in the number of papers published on this topic over the years with most of the observational studies published in the last seven years. Figure 2 shows the distribution of studies according to type of study and year of publication.

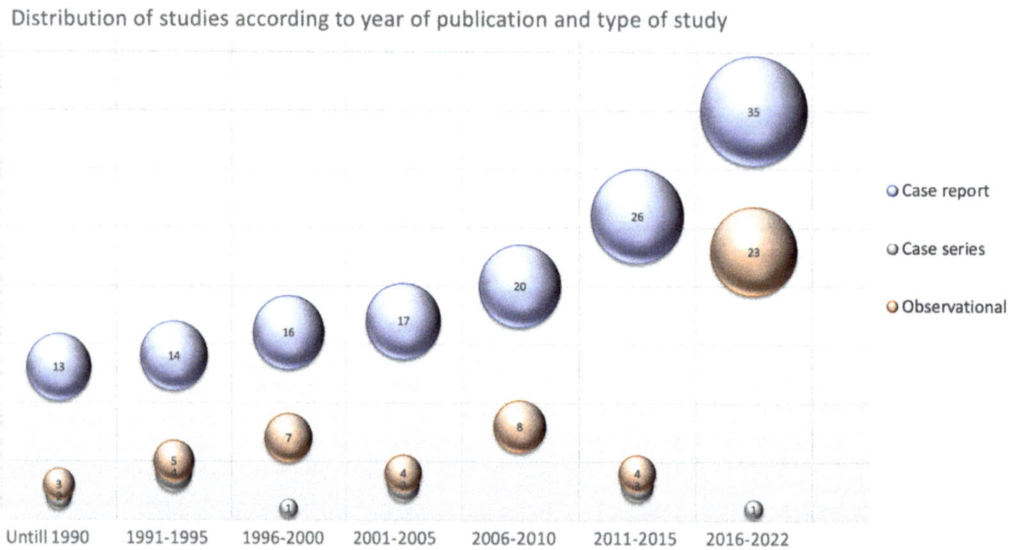

Figure 2. Distribution of studies according to type of study and year of publication.

Most of the papers (141, 67.5%), were case reports, 14 (6.7%) case series, and 54 (25.8%) observational studies. Eighty-seven studies (41.6%) were performed in North America, 60 (28.7%) in Europe, 47 (22.5%) in Asia, and the remaining 15 (7.2%) in Africa or Oceania or Central/South America. In only five studies, a multivariable analysis investigating factors associated with iGAS was performed. The cumulative number of patients in all the studies was 3068 (1222 females, 39.8%) with a mean age of 59.9 (±50.04) months and 1145 patients (37.3%) presented at least one comorbidity.

The most frequently reported therapies were clindamycin (for 594 patients, 19.4%), an antibiotic different from clindamycin (for 1667 patients, 54.3%), and immunoglobulins (for 196 patients, 6.4%). Not all the studies reported data about therapy.

Data about outcomes were collected too, pooled from all studies included, which included overall 3068 patients. Between the different studies, two-hundred and seven patients (6.7%) died from the disease, fifteen children (0.5%) died from other causes, and 169 children (5.5%) presented sequelae (Table 2).

Table 2. Population cumulative characteristics.

	Patients (N = 3068)
Female	1222
Age (months)	
Mean (SD)	59.9 (±50.04)
Comorbidity	1145
Clindamycin in addition to other antibiotics	594
Intravenous immunoglobulin	196
Death from disease	207
Death from other causes	15
Alive with sequelae	169

In Table 3, the main characteristics of the five studies performing multivariable analysis are summarized [11,12,15–17]. None of these studies signaled a positive case of GAS detected before the onset of iGAS. According to the multivariable analysis, the risk factors reported were varicella infection, chronic underlying illness, chickenpox associated with the diagnosis of necrotizing fasciitis, presence of the speC gene in the GAS strain, acetaminophen and ibuprofen use, children nonwhite, living in low-income households, exposition to varicella at home, persistent high fever, having more than one other child in the home, and new use of NSAIDs.

Table 3. Characteristics of the studies with a regression analysis. * Both the analyses were controlled for sex and race; "new use of NSAIDs" (nonsteroidal anti-inflammatory drugs) indicates that a case patient started using NSAIDs in the 2 weeks before illness was diagnosed or that a control participant started using NSAIDs in the 2 weeks before the interview.

Author	Number of iGAS	Inclusion Criteria	Previous or Starting Symptoms or Conditions (Number of Patients)	Associated Factors Detected (Univariate Analysis)	Associated Factors Detected (Multivariable Analysis)	GAS Previously Detected and Not Treated	Therapy before iGAS Insurgence	Death for Disease	Sequelae (Number of Patients)
Minodier P, 2009 [15]	68	-Skin and soft tissue infections -Cardiopulmonary GAS -GAS Nervous system -Sepsis -Other iGAS	-Varicella within a month before iGAS (17)	-Gender female; OR, 0.72 (0.25–2.13) -Mean age ± SD; OR, 0.99 (0.98–1.01) -Recent varicella; OR, 7.5 (2.2–25.6) -Mean temperature ± SD; OR, 1.4 (0.8–2.5) -Mean delay symptoms ± SD; OR, 1.4 (0.9–2.03) -STSS; OR, 12.0 (2.1–6.7) -WBC; OR, 1.0 (1.0–1.0) -Polynuclear cells; OR, 1.0 (1.0–1.0) -Lymphocytes; OR, 1.0 (1.0–1.0) -PLT; OR, 1.0 (1.0–1.0) -CRP; OR, 0.99 (0.8–1.0) -GAS positive BC; OR, 0.08 (0.2–0.3) -emm 1 type; OR, 0.4 (0.1–1.5) -Virulence genes speA (OR, 0.4 (0.1–1.5)); speC (OR, 4.7 (1.5–14.7)); ssa (OR, 1.1 (0.3–4.2)); smeZ-1 (OR, 0.4 (0.1–1.5)); sic OR, 0.5 (0.1–1.8)	**-Varicella infection (OR, 6.2; 95% CI, 1.7–22.4)** **-Presence of *speC* gene in GAS strain (OR, 4.0; 95% CI, 1.2–13.9)**	Not specified	Not specified	3	Not specified
Stefanie Gauguet, 2015 [16]	86	-Sepsis -STSS -Skin and soft tissue	-Varicella (15) -Pharyngitis (13) -Other skin lesions (7) -Otitis media (4) -Sinusitis (2) -Central venous catheter infection (2) -Surgical wound infection (1)	-Comorbid illness; OR, 1.01 (0.35–2.87) -Immunosuppression; OR, 0.38 (0.08–1.82)	-Bacteriemia without a source. Adjusted OR, 0.08 (0.01–0.67)	Not specified	Not specified	2	Amputation (8)

Table 3. *Cont.*

Author	Number of iGAS	Inclusion Criteria	Previous or Starting Symptoms or Conditions (Number of Patients)	Associated Factors Detected (Univariate Analysis)	Associated Factors Detected (Multivariable Analysis)	GAS Previously Detected and Not Treated	Therapy before iGAS Insurgence	Death for Disease	Sequelae (Number of Patients)
Kevin B. Laupland, 2000 [12]	243	-Skin and soft tissue -Cardiopulmonary iGAS -GAS Nervous system -Sepsis -Osteomyelitis iGAS	-Varicella (31) -Asthma (12) -Malignancy (11) -Congenital cardiac disease (4) -Biliary atresia (3) -Juvenile rheumatoid arthritis (1) -Dermatomyositis (1) -Renal transplant (1) -Seizure disorder (1) -Ependymoma of brainstem (1) -Quadriplegia (1) -Cerebral palsy (1) -Multiple congenital anomalies (1)	-Leukemia; RR, 44 (30–56) -Asthma; RR, 0.74 (0.42–1.33) -Antecedent chickenpox associated with diagnosis of necrotizing fasciitis; RR, 6.3 (1.8–22.3)	**-Chronic underlying illness; RR, 11 (2.4–45)** **-Chickenpox associated with the diagnosis of necrotizing fasciitis (for the subset of children with soft tissue infection); RR, 4.5 (1.0–20)**	Not specified	Not specified	3	0
Samuel M. Lesko, 2001 [17]	52	-iGAS -Skin and soft tissue infection	-Varicella (52)	-Acetaminophen only use; OR, 0.96 (0.43–2.2) -Ibuprofen only use; OR, 1.5 (0.44–5.1) -Both (acetaminophen and ibuprofen); OR, 5.0 (1.6–16)	-Acetaminophen only use; OR, 0.94 (0.34–2.6) -Ibuprofen only use; OR, 2.5 (0.58–11) **-Both (acetaminophen and ibuprofen); OR, 5.6 (1.2–25)** **-Children nonwhite; OR, 3.8, (1.4–11)** **-Children living in low-income households; OR, 5.1 (1.7–15)** **-Exposed to varicella at home; OR, 6.4 (2.6–16)** **-Persistent high fever; OR, 9.6 (2.8–33).** -Use of ibuprofen before the development of signs or symptoms of this complication; OR, 1.3 (0.33–5.3)	Not specified	-Acetaminophen only, for Varicella symptoms (19) -Ibuprofen only (5) -Acetaminophen and ibuprofen (13)	0	0

Table 3. *Cont.*

Author	Number of iGAS	Inclusion Criteria	Previous or Starting Symptoms or Conditions (Number of Patients)	Associated Factors Detected (Univariate Analysis)	Associated Factors Detected (Multivariable Analysis)	GAS Previously Detected and Not Treated	Therapy before iGAS Insurgence	Death for Disease	Sequelae (Number of Patients)
Factor SH, 2005 [11]	38	iGAS	-VZV infection (3 patients) -HIV infection (1 patient)	* -Having a primary caretaker who smokes; OR, 2.71 (1.02–7.21) -Presence of >1 other child in the home; OR, 5.76 (1.95–16.96) -New use of NSAIDs; OR, 3.15 (1.07–9.29) -More rooms in the home; OR, 0.81 (0.66–0.99) -Higher level of parental education; OR, 0.69 (0.51–0.91) -A household member with a runny nose (rhinitis) in the past 2 weeks; OR, 0.25 (0.08–0.80)	*** -Having >1 other child in the home; OR, 16.85 (3.9–72.84)** **-//new use of nonsteroidal anti-inflammatory drugs (NSAIDs); OR, 10.64 (2.08–54.61)** -More rooms in the home; OR, 0.67 (0.51–0.88) -Having a household member with a runny nose in the past 2 weeks; OR, 0.09 (0.01–0.4)	Not specified	-NSAIDs (9 patients) -Steroids (1 patient)	2	Not specified

4. Discussion

In this scoping review, we analyzed the existing literature, providing information on the risk factors, localizations, treatments, and outcomes of children with iGAS. In particular, our focus was to address if studies explored risk factors for iGAS, including common symptoms like pharyngitis/otitis and whether previous GAS infections and whether antibiotics were associated with the development of iGAS. Unfortunately, we found only five well-designed studies that could provide multivariate analyses on risk factors associated with iGAS, and no studies provided information about previous infection/colonization with GAS in children later diagnosed with iGAS, nor was information available about any antibiotic treatment of a potential prodromal phase of iGAS. In addition, no randomized controlled trials were found that explored the role of IVIG, in association or not in association with clindamycin, on the outcomes of iGAS. Our study, therefore, highlights important gaps in current knowledge which is reflected in the uncertainty of medical doctors about what to do to prevent iGAS infection. To our knowledge, this is the first systematic mapping, through a standardized scoping review approach based on PRISMA guidelines, of all available works in the literature on risk factors and treatments used for iGAS, including details about types of study. In particular, the strongest risk factors highlighted in the studies with multivariable analysis were varicella infection (OR, 6.2; 95% CI, 1.7–22.4) in the Minodier study [15]; association with the diagnosis of necrotizing fasciitis (RR, 4.5 (1.0–20)) in the Laupland study [12]; exposure to varicella (OR 6.4 (2.6–16)) in the Lesko study [17]); presence of the speC gene in GAS strains (OR, 4.0; 95% CI, 1.2–13.9) [15]; acetaminophen and ibuprofen use (according to Lesko [17], acetaminophen only use (OR, 0.94 (0.34–2.6)), ibuprofen only use (OR, 2.5 (0.58–11)), and both (acetaminophen and ibuprofen) (OR 5.6 (1.2–25)); according to Factor [11], (NSAIDs) OR, 10.64 (2.08–54.61)); children nonwhite; living in low-income households; exposure to varicella at home; persistent high fever; having more than one other child in the home; and new use of nonsteroidal anti-inflammatory drugs (NSAIDs) [11,12]. These data are mostly in line with previous publications in the literature describing that the presence of one other child living in the same house, varicella zoster virus infection, and the use of nonsteroidal anti-inflammatory drugs have been reported in the literature as risk factors for iGAS [11,12]. Of the five studies performing multivariate analyses and including a total of 487 children, details about the diagnosis of pharyngitis, otitis, or sinusitis before iGAS were reported only for 13, 4, and 2 children, respectively, and it was not clear for any of them if they were tested or not for GAS. This means that, in 2023, we are still unaware if a diagnosis of iGAS is preceded by a non-invasive infection (or colonization) with GAS and, as a consequence, it is completely unknown if low thresholds for testing and treating GAS may have any effect on reducing iGAS incidence, even in periods of high numbers of cases, as may happen in cold seasons with high circulation of respiratory viruses. As such, at the moment, clinicians should not test every child with mild symptoms or non-consistent symptoms for GAS nor routinely offer empiric treatment with penicillin or beta-lactams in an attempt to prevent iGAS. Similarly, such information should be transferred to the public in order to avoid the exaggerated fear of iGAS noticed during the 2022–23 winter season in Europe, which may have worse longer-term implications such as antibiotic shortages, development of drug resistance, and an overflow of patients in emergency departments. With the limited current state of knowledge, it is plausible that indiscriminate GAS testing and treatment may have a minimal effect in preventing iGAS infections.

To better understand if children with iGAS have, in the days or weeks before the disease, a possible GAS infection/colonization that might have been diagnosed and treated to prevent iGAS, new prospective studies are highly needed. In this regard, a new European pediatric prospective study (PEGASUS) is currently implementing an observational study on pediatric invasive group A streptococcal disease, with the aim of describing the incidence, risk factors, clinical phenotypes, microbiology and resistance, treatment, and outcomes of iGAS in children across Europe (https://www.pegasus-study.eu/, accessed on 20 July 2023).

Although our scoping review highlights that no studies investigated what happened in the weeks before the diagnosis of iGAS, the reinforcement that chickenpox is a strong risk factor in several studies may have public health implications. For example, some countries like United Kingdom do not routinely suggest chickenpox vaccination for children [18] for several reasons, including the usual self-limiting nature of the illness and the possible faster decline in induced immunity compared with natural immunity, which in turn can predispose zoster and other VZV complications in the elderly population [19]. However, considering the high burden of iGAS in countries like the UK and its association with previous cases of chickenpox, such a choice may be reconsidered (if not, the public should at least be made aware of this association and possible indirect benefit of the vaccination) to provide a more comprehensive decision to parents [20,21].

In this scoping, we mapped the therapeutic strategies used to manage iGAS infection. Currently, most guidelines do not give strong indications about the use of clindamycin and/or IVIG, although most experts use them. Clindamycin is a frequent choice given its action of ribosome and the consequent ability to inhibit protein synthesis, therefore limiting the production of GAS toxins [22]. Similarly, IVIG can neutralize toxin activity [23]. However, none of the studies that used clindamycin or IVIG were randomized or randomized controlled trials. As such, even a systematic review or meta-analysis to reply to this question would not be enough, while a RCT to understand the role of clindamycin, with or without IVIG, is highly needed. Currently, the ability to link multinational referral centers should allow such a study design. Of note, a recent Japanese nationwide observational study evaluated the effectiveness of intravenous immunoglobulin therapy for invasive group A Streptococcus infection [24]. A total of 481 patients (median age, 65 years; female, 49.7%) were included in the analysis. The overall mortality rate was 31.0%. After adjusting for background factors, we found that IVIG treatment had no effect on in-hospital mortality (adjusted odds ratio (OR): 0.99, 95% confidence interval (CI): 0.93–1.04, $p = 0.92$). Similar results were obtained after propensity score matching (OR: 1.00, 95% CI: 0.62–1.61, $p > 0.99$). The authors concluded that IVIG administration had no survival benefit in adult iGAS patients.

An important finding of this paper is the underrepresentation of iGAS publications from low-to-middle-income countries (LMICs). Paradoxically, LMICs are the countries that still suffer the most from non-suppurative consequences of GAS infections, including rheumatic fever [25]. Therefore, it is plausible to expect that these countries also have a higher incidence of GAS and iGAS infections, particularly if we consider that, in our scoping review, being of nonwhite ethnicity was also a risk factor in developing iGAS. This represents an important gap and this information should be used by policy makers and funding agencies to facilitate multinational studies on the topic that also include LMICs.

All together, the findings of our scoping review, despite highlighting current gaps in iGAS knowledge, may still provide some recommendations to healthcare professionals. First, we were not able to find studies evaluating whether iGAS is the consequence of an unrecognized uncomplicated GAS infection and, therefore, indiscriminate use of antibiotics in any tonsillitis case is not appropriate. However, some strong risk factors are coherent in several studies, such as previous cases of chickenpox. Therefore, a possible strategy for next winter to limit iGAS cases, in light of the unexpectedly high peak cases of 2022–2023, would be to expand the access to varicella vaccinations in children in those countries not recommending it. In a survey performed in the Netherlands, varicella infection preceded all cases of necrotizing fasciitis [26]. In the Netherlands, varicella vaccination is not included in the national immunization program and the 2022 varicella epidemic in the Netherlands was higher than expected, leading the authors to speculate if varicella infections contributed to recent surges of iGAS [27]. In periods of high GAS circulation and notification of iGAS cases, like in the current post-pandemic era, a rethinking of the indirect benefits of varicella vaccination on iGAS development may be warranted. Also, two studies [11,17] found an association of NSAIDs, confirmed by an older review as well [28]. Although a causative link has not been proven, hypotheses for such an effect have been proposed, including the ability of NSAIDs to interrupt the negative feedback loop that limits production of tumor necrosis factor (TNF)-alpha or its possible role in masking the signs and symptoms of developing severe infection [29,30]. As such, healthcare professionals and public policy makers may consider providing balanced information campaigns on the use of over-the-counter medications for pain and fever to the public, particularly in periods of high GAS circulation and unusual increase in notification rates of iGAS cases.

Our scoping review has some limitations. We only included studies published in English. Although we also attempted a mixed approach linking a mapping of the literature with a synthesis of main data when feasible, we did not perform a meta-analyses and sensitivity data reported should be considered as approximate to provide a general perspective of what is known on the topic. Also, our search was limited to the two databases SCOPUS and Pubmed. Although this is a limitation, we still screened as many as 4198 papers, and two is the minimum required numbers of databases for systematic reviews, and we only had access to them in our institution. Last, the article extraction process was performed by two authors due to the extensive number of articles, an approach that carries the potential for bias, although the two reviewers were trained on data extraction by the PI (DB) and the coordinator of the search strategy (FM).

5. Conclusions

In conclusion, our scoping review highlights important gaps on several aspects of iGAS in children, including prodromic presentation and optimal treatment strategies. No pediatric trials were found, and only a small number of studies have been performed in LMICs, where iGAS may have a higher incidence. Only four studies were prospective. Our findings should inform researchers, policy makers and funding agencies on which study designs should be prioritized on this topic, focusing efforts and funds on those studies that may help us in responding the most important questions on this topic: researchers have to better understand how we can recognize, and treat, early GAS infections to prevent the development of iGAS and clarify if the use of clindamycin, with or without IVIG, improves outcomes of iGAS.

Supplementary Materials: The following supporting information can be downloaded at: https://www.mdpi.com/article/10.3390/children10091472/s1.

Author Contributions: Conceptualization, D.B. and P.V.; methodology, F.M.; formal analysis, F.M.; investigation, C.G., V.P. and L.M.; data curation, D.B. and F.M.; writing—original draft preparation, D.B., F.M. and L.M.; writing—review and editing, D.B. and P.V.; supervision, P.V. All authors have read and agreed to the published version of the manuscript.

Funding: This research received no external funding.

Institutional Review Board Statement: Not applicable.

Informed Consent Statement: Not applicable.

Data Availability Statement: Dataset available upon request to the corresponding author.

Conflicts of Interest: The authors declare no conflict of interest.

References

1. Steer, A.C.; Lamagni, T.; Curtis, N.; Carapetis, J.R. Invasive group a streptococcal disease: Epidemiology, pathogenesis and management. *Drugs* **2012**, *72*, 1213–1227. [CrossRef]
2. Ma, C.; Gao, X.; Wu, S.; Zhang, L.; Wang, J.; Zhang, Z.; Yao, Z.; Song, X.; Li, W.; Wang, X.; et al. M Protein of Group a Streptococcus Plays an Essential Role in Inducing High Expression of A20 in Macrophages Resulting in the Downregulation of Inflammatory Response in Lung Tissue. *Front. Cell. Infect. Microbiol.* **2018**, *8*, 131. [CrossRef]
3. Frost, H.R.; Sanderson-Smith, M.; Walker, M.; Botteaux, A.; Smeesters, P.R. Group A streptococcal M-like proteins: From pathogenesis to vaccine potential. *FEMS Microbiol. Rev.* **2018**, *42*, 193–204. [CrossRef]
4. Available online: https://www.cdc.gov/abcs/reports-findings/data-2020.html (accessed on 1 May 2023).
5. Available online: https://emergency.cdc.gov/han/2022/han00484.asp (accessed on 1 May 2023).

6. Available online: https://www.ecdc.europa.eu/en/news-events/increase-invasive-group-streptococcal-infections-among-children-europe-including (accessed on 1 May 2023).
7. de Gier, B.; Marchal, N.; de Beer-Schuurman, I.; Te Wierik, M.; Hooiveld, M.; ISIS-AR Study Group; GAS Study Group; de Melker, H.E.; van Sorge, N.M. Increase in invasive group A streptococcal (*Streptococcus pyogenes*) infections (iGAS) in young children in The Netherlands, 2022. *Eurosurveillance* **2023**, *28*, 2200941. [CrossRef] [PubMed]
8. Guy, R.; Henderson, K.L.; Coelho, J.; Hughes, H.; Mason, E.L.; Gerver, S.M.; Demirjian, A.; Watson, C.; Sharp, A.; Brown, C.S.; et al. Increase in invasive group A streptococcal infection notifications, England, 2022. *Eurosurveillance* **2023**, *28*, 2200942. [CrossRef] [PubMed]
9. Available online: https://www.who.int/emergencies/disease-outbreak-news/item/2022-DON429 (accessed on 1 May 2023).
10. Available online: https://www.ema.europa.eu/en/documents/shortage/amoxicillin-amoxicillin/clavulanic-acid-supply-shortage_en.pdf (accessed on 1 July 2023).
11. Factor, S.H.; Levine, O.S.; Harrison, L.H.; Farley, M.M.; McGeer, A.; Skoff, T.; Wright, C.; Schwartz, B.; Schuchat, A. Risk factors for pediatric invasive group A streptococcal disease. *Emerg. Infect. Dis.* **2005**, *11*, 1062–1066. [CrossRef] [PubMed]
12. Laupland, K.B.; Davies, H.D.; Low, D.E.; Schwartz, B.; Green, K.; McGeer, A. Invasive group A streptococcal disease in children and association with varicella-zoster virus infection. Ontario Group A Streptococcal Study Group. *Pediatrics* **2020**, *105*, E60. [CrossRef]
13. Mariani, F.; Martino, L.; Gentili, C.; Pulcinelli, V.; Valentini, P.; Buonsenso, D. State-of-the-art of invasive Group A Streptococcus infection in children: Protocol for a scoping review of the literature with a focus on predictors of invasive infection [version 1; peer review: 1 approved]. *F1000Research* **2023**, *12*, 209. [CrossRef]
14. Tricco, A.C.; Lillie, E.; Zarin, W.; O'Brien, K.K.; Colquhoun, H.; Levac, D.; Moher, D.; Peters, M.D.J.; Horsley, T.; Weeks, L.; et al. PRISMA Extension for Scoping Reviews (PRISMA-ScR): Checklist and Explanation. *Ann. Intern. Med.* **2018**, *169*, 467–473. [CrossRef]
15. Minodier, P.; Bidet, P.; Rallu, F.; Tapiero, B.; Bingen, E.; Ovetchkine, P. Clinical and microbiologic characteristics of group A streptococcal necrotizing fasciitis in children. *Pediatr. Infect. Dis. J.* **2009**, *28*, 541–543. [CrossRef]
16. Gauguet, S.; Ahmed, A.A.; Zhou, J.; Pfoh, E.R.; Ahnger-Pier, K.K.; Harper, M.B.; Ozonoff, A.; Wessels, M.R.; Lee, G.M. Group A streptococcal bacteremia without a source is associated with less severe disease in children. *Pediatr. Infect. Dis. J.* **2015**, *34*, 447–449. [CrossRef]
17. Lesko, S.M.; O'Brien, K.L.; Schwartz, B.; Vezina, R.; Mitchell, A.A. Invasive group A streptococcal infection and nonsteroidal antiinflammatory drug use among children with primary varicella. *Pediatrics* **2001**, *107*, 1108–1115. [CrossRef] [PubMed]
18. Available online: https://www.nhs.uk/conditions/vaccinations/chickenpox-vaccine/ (accessed on 1 July 2023).
19. Marin, M.; Seward, J.F.; Gershon, A.A. 25 Years of Varicella Vaccination in the United States. *J. Infect. Dis.* **2022**, *226* (Suppl. S4), S375–S379. [CrossRef] [PubMed]
20. Available online: https://www.bloomberg.com/news/articles/2023-04-24/uk-moves-toward-embracing-chickenpox-vaccine-in-policy-reversal (accessed on 1 July 2023).
21. Sherman, S.M.; Lingley-Heath, N.; Lai, J.; Sim, J.; Bedford, H. Parental acceptance of and preferences for administration of routine varicella vaccination in the UK: A study to inform policy. *Vaccine* **2023**, *41*, 1438–1446. [CrossRef] [PubMed]
22. Azeh, I.; Gerber, J.; Wellmer, A.; Wellhausen, M.; Koenig, B.; Eiffert, H.; Nau, R. Protein synthesis inhibiting clindamycin improves outcome in a mouse model of Staphylococcus aureus sepsis compared with the cell wall active ceftriaxone. *Crit. Care Med.* **2002**, *30*, 1560–1564. [CrossRef]
23. Amreen, S.; Brar, S.K.; Perveen, S.; Chaudhry, M.R.; AlBabtain, S.; Khan, S. Clinical Efficacy of Intravenous Immunoglobulins in Management of Toxic Shock Syndrome: An Updated Literature Review. *Cureus* **2021**, *13*, e12836. [CrossRef]
24. Senda, A.; Endo, A.; Fushimi, K.; Otomo, Y. Effectiveness of Intravenous Immunoglobulin Therapy for Invasive Group A Streptococcus Infection: A Japanese Nationwide Observational Study. *Int. J. Infect. Dis.* **2023**. *ahead of print*. [CrossRef]
25. Barth, D.D.; Naicker, P.; Engel, K.; Muhamed, B.; Basera, W.; Mayosi, B.M.; Dale, J.B.; Engel, M.E. Molecular Epidemiology of Noninvasive and Invasive Group A Streptococcal Infections in Cape Town. *mSphere* **2019**, *4*, e00421-19. [CrossRef]
26. van Kempen, E.B.; Bruijning-Verhagen, P.C.J.; Borensztajn, D.; Vermont, C.L.; Quaak, M.S.W.; Janson, J.A.; Maat, I.; Stol, K.; Vlaminckx, B.J.M.; Wieringa, J.W.; et al. Increase in Invasive Group a Streptococcal Infections in Children in the Netherlands, A Survey Among 7 Hospitals in 2022. *Pediatr. Infect. Dis. J.* **2023**, *42*, e122–e124. [CrossRef]
27. Netherlands Institute for Health Services Research (NIVEL). Communication: Increase in Chicken-Pox in Children Possible Catch-Up Effect after Coronayears ("Toename Waterpokken Bij Kinderen Mogelijk Inhaaleffect na Coronajaren"). 2022. Available online: https://www.nivel.nl/nl/nieuws/toename-waterpokken-bij-kinderen-mogelijk-inhaaleffect-na-coronajaren (accessed on 7 December 2022).
28. Hamilton, S.M.; Bayer, C.R.; Stevens, D.L.; Bryant, A.E. Effects of selective and nonselective nonsteroidal anti-inflammatory drugs on antibiotic efficacy of experimental group A streptococcal myonecrosis. *J. Infect. Dis.* **2014**, *209*, 1429–1435. [CrossRef]

29. Bryant, A.E.; Bayer, C.R.; Aldape, M.J.; Stevens, D.L. The roles of injury and nonsteroidal anti-inflammatory drugs in the development and outcomes of severe group A streptococcal soft tissue infections. *Curr. Opin. Infect. Dis.* **2015**, *28*, 231–239. [CrossRef] [PubMed]
30. Ture, Z.; Demiraslan, H.; Kontas, O.; Alp, E.; Doganay, M. The role of nonsteroidal anti-inflammatory drugs intramuscular injection in the development and severity of deep soft tissue infection in mice. *Fundam. Clin. Pharmacol.* **2018**, *32*, 147–154. [CrossRef] [PubMed]

children

MDPI

Case Report

Toxic Streptococcal Infection in Children: Report on Two Cases with Uncharacteristic Course of Scarlet Fever

Krystyna Stencel-Gabriel [1], Dawid Konwant [1,2,*] and Karolina Szejnoga-Tułacz [1]

1 Department of Pediatrics, Faculty of Health Sciences in Katowice, Medical University of Silesia in Katowice, 40-055 Katowice, Poland
2 Doctoral School, Medical University of Silesia in Katowice, 40-055 Katowice, Poland
* Correspondence: dawid.konwant@med.sum.edu.pl

Abstract: Introduction: Scarlet fever is usually a mild childhood disease caused by type A *streptococci*. This disease is spread by droplets, mainly through direct contact with an infected person or the objects they have used. In pediatrics, these are significant risk factors for the transmission of infectious diseases. However, it is important to remember the possibility of serious complications in the course of scarlet fever. Aim: This paper provides a discussion of two pediatric cases in order to determine the possibilities of diagnosis, differentiation, and treatment of patients with severe, non-obvious courses of scarlet fever. Methods: The case reports of two patients hospitalized in a pediatric department due to *Streptococcus pyogenes* infection were examined. Results: The patients were admitted to the emergency room with symptoms not directly indicative of type A streptococcal infection, which required further diagnosis. Both patients complained of weakness at the time of presentation. They had an elevated temperature, were dehydrated during the course of gastroenteritis, and passed liquid stools without pathological admixtures. Further stages of diagnosis and treatment required hospitalization in the pediatric department. Therapeutic benefit from the implemented treatment was obtained, and the patients were discharged in good general condition with further recommendations. Conclusions: Medical history, which is often very detailed, can be the key to making the final diagnosis and can supplement the data collected on the basis of laboratory tests. Scarlet fever does not always occur with a mild course, and sometimes its course can be quite non-specific and may require a thorough diagnosis.

Keywords: streptococcal infection; children; scarlet fever; hospitalization

1. Introduction

Streptococcus pyogenes is a bacterium belonging to group A *streptococci* (GAS), which is a significant etiological factor of infections in children, but also among adults. This pathogen causes a number of infections in the pediatric population, including pharyngitis, tonsillitis, scarlet fever, infectious impetigo, pneumonia or subcutaneous tissue inflammation, erysipelas, and toxic shock syndrome. Pharyngitis is one of the milder forms of infection, with approximately 616 million cases diagnosed worldwide each year. Existing statistical data indicate that there are about 163 thousand deaths annually in the world due to invasive streptococcal infection. Thus, it is an important epidemiological risk factor for death and severe complications [1]. Scarlet fever is a common infectious disease with a characteristic morphology; however, according to existing data, its diagnosis is often delayed or not considered at all in groups of children over five years of age due to its similarity to streptococcal pharyngitis [2,3]. Distinguishing between viral and bacterial etiologies of acute pharyngitis can be problematic when attempting to make a correct diagnosis. Current statistics indicate that for acute pharyngitis and acute tonsillitis in children, less than 30% are of bacterial origin [4,5]. The highest peak incidence of GAS pharyngitis is observed during winter months. In addition, an increased number of cases may also occur in spring and summer [4,6].

This paper presents two cases of patients hospitalized in the Department of Pediatrics, Medical University of Silesia, in which the medical interview turned out to be the key to making the final diagnosis of severe, atypical scarlet fever.

2. Case Reports

2.1. Patient 1

2.1.1. Patient Information

A 4-year-old patient came to the emergency room in the Department of Pediatrics due to dehydration during the course of gastroenteritis and worsening skin lesions. Over the previous three days before admission, the boy had a high and intense fever reaching 41 °C with a mediocre response to antipyretics. He passed numerous liquid stools without pathological admixtures. On the day before hospital admission, a small, maculopapular, and itchy rash was present on the patient's skin, as well as redness. His lips were dry and cracked. The boy drank water quite willingly, but his diuresis was significantly limited according to his parents' opinion. The examination showed that the patient and his parents had an upper respiratory tract infection two months before hospitalization, when he received Cefuroxime orally in a dose appropriate for his age. Subsequently, three weeks before hospitalization in the ward, the patient received Clarithromycin in the oral form for 14 days as an outpatient due to pharyngitis. The information obtained from the parents did not indicate that the patient had contracted COVID-19.

2.1.2. Clinical Findings and Diagnostic Assessment

In the emergency room, a physical examination revealed severe signs of dehydration, an average clinical condition, significant weakness (the appearance of a very sick child), and discrete swelling of the hands and feet. Moreover, the patient had chapped redness of the lips, with swelling of the gums and tongue, and cervical lymphadenopathy with predominance on the left side. The patient's skin showed erythema on the face, and fine-petal rash in the area of the chest, abdomen, back, and buttocks.

The preliminary laboratory tests showed high inflammatory parameters, leukocytosis with neutrophilia, hyponatremia, compensated metabolic acidosis, high urea concentration, and decreased GFR (Table 1). Initially, due to the child's severe clinical condition and significantly elevated inflammatory parameters, which could indicate severe sepsis, cultures were taken from urine (negative result), feces (negative result), blood (negative result), and from a throat swab. The quantitative test for antibodies on the second day of his stay turned out to be positive, with a result of 141.2 U/mL. During hospitalization, it was hypothesized that the patient might have contracted COVID-19 during the infection two months prior to admission to the ward. Control laboratory tests, including inflammatory parameters, were performed after 72 and 96 h of hospitalization and at the end of therapy, i.e., on the nineth day of therapy (Table 2). On the fifth day, the result of the microbiological examination of the throat was obtained, which showed the presence of *streptococcus pyogenes* in the high titer (++). This bacterial species is sensitive to beta-lactam antibiotics. Thus, penicillin was the drug of choice. During hospitalization, abdominal ultrasound was performed four times, lung ultrasound was performed three times, and lymph node ultrasound was performed once. The first ultrasound examination of the abdominal cavity performed on the second day of hospitalization showed a slight amount of interloop fluid. In the next two follow-up examinations which were carried out on consecutive days, there was no deterioration. The last follow-up examination performed on the 9th day of hospitalization showed a regression of the previously described changes. The first ultrasound of the lungs was performed on the second day of treatment, showing slight bilateral inflammatory consolidations at the bottom of the lungs, which was confirmed in the next ultrasound imaging performed 24 h later, resulting in the diagnosis of bilateral pneumonia in the child. The examination performed on the nineth day of treatment confirmed the regression of the previously described inflammatory changes in the lungs. The cervical and submandibular lymph node examination on the fourth day showed inflammatory lymphadenopathy.

The patient was consulted twice by a cardiologist on the third and tenth days of treatment due to his severe general condition during the initial days of hospitalization. The performed electrocardiographic and echocardiographic examinations showed no significant abnormalities. Despite this, the consulting cardiologist additionally recommended using NT-proBNP, cardiac markers, and daily monitoring of electrocardiogram for the purpose of differential diagnosis of pediatric inflammatory multisystem syndrome temporally associated with SARS-CoV-2 (PIMS-TS). Laryngological consultation was carried out on the third day of hospitalization, during which a strongly reddened throat and swollen purulent deposits on the tonsils were found.

Table 1. Initial diagnosis in the emergency room.

Marked Laboratory Tests	Patient Number 1	Patient Number 2	Normal Ranges
	Complete blood count		
WBC [$\times 10^3/\mu L$ (%)]	17.9	10.6	[4.0–10.0]
Neut [$\times 10^3/\mu L$ (%)]	15.6 (87.2%)	8.4 (79.8%)	[1.2–6.0]
Lymph [$\times 10^3/\mu L$ (%)]	0.4 (2.4%)	0.6 (5.4%)	[1.0–5.5]
Mono [$\times 10^3/\mu L$ (%)]	1.4 (7.9%)	1.2 (11.6%)	[−1.0]
Eosy [$\times 10^3/\mu L$ (%)]	0.2 (1.1%)	0.1 (1.0%)	[−0.7]
Baos [$\times 10^3/\mu L$ (%)]	0.3 (1.5%)	0.2 (2.2%)	[−0.1]
RBC [$\times 10^6/\mu L$]	4.47	4.25	[4.0–5.3]
Hgb [g/dL]	12.5	12.0	[11.5–14.5]
HCT [%]	35.2	34.3	[33.0–43.0]
MCV [fL]	78.7	80.6	[76.0–90.0]
MCH [pg]	27.9	28.2	[25.0–31.0]
MCHC [g/dL]	35.5	35.1	[32.0–36.0]
Rdw [%]	11.3	10.2	[10.0–14.5]
PLT [$\times 10^3/\mu L$]	322	276	[150–400]
MPV [fl]	5.4	5.5	[5.5–12.2]
CRP [mg/L]	290.68	165.7	[−5.0]
Procalcitonin [ng/mL]	51.6	5.0	[−0.5]
ALT [U/L]	37.5	196.3	[−41.0]
AST [U/L]	51.9	173.9	[−41.0]
Urea [mg/dL]	55.9	38.1	[16.6–48.5]
Creatinine [mg/dL]	0.61	0.57	[0.7–1.2]
GFR [mL/min]	51	56.3	[>60]
Sodium [mmol/L]	130	131	[135–145]
Potassium [mmol/L]	4.41	3.66	[3.5–5.1]
	Capillary blood gases		
pH	7.40	7.42	[7.3–7.4]
pCO2 [mmHg]	26.2	33.7	[35.0–45.0]
O2 [mmHg]	61.6	73.5	[65.0–100.0]
BE	−8.6	−2.9	[−2–+2]
	General examination of urine		
		Cloudy urine	
Color	Cloudy urine	5–10 HPF	Light yellow color
Leukocytes	0–2 HPF	-	<5 HPF
Ketone bodies	++	2–4 HPF	-
RBCs	-	Single hyaline cast HPF	-
		Single bacteria HPF	

Abbreviations: WBC—white blood count total; Neut—neutrophils total; Limf—total lymphocytes; Mono—monocytes; Eosy—eosinophils; Baso—basophils; RBC—total red blood count; Hgb—hemoglobin concentration; Hct—hematocrit; MCV—mean corpuscular volume; MCH—mean corpuscular hemoglobin; MCHC—mean corpuscular hemoglobin concentration; Rdw—red blood cell distribution width; Plt—total platelet count; MPV—mean platelet volume; and RBCs—red blood cells.

Table 2. Diagnostics during hospitalization in the Department of Pediatrics.

Marked Laboratory Tests	I Control		II Control		III Control	
	Patient Number 1 (3rd Day of Hospitalization)	Patient Number 2 (2nd Day of Hospitalization)	Patient Number 1 (4th Day of Hospitalization)	Patient Number 2 (4th Day of Hospitalization)	Patient Number 1 (9th Day of Hospitalization)	Patient Number 2 (10th Day of Hospitalization)
Complete blood count						
WBC [$\times 10^3/\mu L$ (%)]	17.7	9.7	14.1	10.4	18.2	10.6
Neut [$\times 10^3/\mu L$ (%)]	9.1	6.0 (61.7%)	3.8 (26.6%)	4.5 (43.4%)	11.8 (65.1%)	5.2 (49.0%)
Hgb [g/dL]	11.1	10.9 g/dL	11.2	10.61	12.61	12.4
PLT [$\times 10^3/\mu L$]	181	226	152	243	412	514
CRP [mg/L]	178.7	103.86	87.45	71.4	43.9	39.0
PCT [ng/mL]	18.8	2.2	6.7	1.8	3.3	0.5
ALT [U/L]	33.9	116.3	32.7	90.5	33.8	77.2
AST [U/L]	40.4	53.6	32.9	48.3	36.6	44.4
Creatinine [mg/dL]	<0.4	0.38	0.24	0.39	0.24	0.33
GFR [mL/min]	79.9	84.5	129.8	82.3	129.8	97.3
Urea [mg/dL]	30.1	22.4	20.1	23.1	18.6	23.0
Total protein [g/dL]	5.59	5.02	5.46	5.21	5.69	7.68
Total cholesterol [mg/dL]	99	140	101	204	172	180
Triglycerides [mg/dL]	307	492	338	442	342	223
LDL fraction [mg/dL]	9	13	10	22	118	150
HDL fraction [mg/dL]	14	14	13	12	23	36
Fibrinogen [g/L]	4.9	4.6	2.7	3.0	2.1	2.5
APTT [sec]	27	31	26	29	29	27
INR	0.9	1.2	1.0	1.1	1.0	1.0
D-dimer [mg//]	1.6	1.14	1.9	5.19	0.8	0.7
Troponin T [pg/mL]	4.9	4.7	4.8	4.8	4.7	4.4
CK-MB [U/L]	20.4	19.6	23.6	21.5	19.8	21.9
NT-proBNP	1178	995	-	-	425	-
Albumin [g/dL]	3.14	2.9	-	-	3.0	-

Abbreviations: WBC—total white blood count total; Neut—total neutrophils; Hgb—hemoglobin concentration; Plt—total platelet count; and MPV—mean platelet volume. I Control refers to laboratory tests performed between 24 and 48 h of hospitalization. II Control refers to tests performed again on the 4th day of hospitalization. III Control refers to tests performed at the final stage of hospitalization on day 9 or 10.

2.1.3. Therapeutic Interventions and Outcome

On the first day of hospitalization, after the laboratory tests, Ceftriaxone at 50 mg/kg/day in the intravenous form was introduced to the treatment, and after the next three days, 10 mg/kg/dose of Vancomycin was also added and administered intravenously four times a day. This drug was implemented due to the lack of improvement after the treatment used so far. It was suspected, due to the lack of a definitive throat swab, that a penicillin-resistant pathogen might be the source of the infection. After the use of third-generation cephalosporin, laboratory tests showed a decrease in inflammatory parameters (Table 2), but the boy's clinical condition did not improve. In addition, diuresis was limited

(400 mL per 24 h). There was swelling of the feet, hands, and the lumbosacral area. The erythematous rash persisted. Apart from pharyngitis and tonsillitis, extensive stomatitis developed in the oral cavity, which prevented the patient from taking liquids and food.

Based on a positive throat swab obtained on day 5 of hospitalization, the patient was diagnosed with scarlet fever. *Streptococcus pyogenes* was grown to a large extent, as well as *Haemophilus parainfluenzae*. On the same day, oral Phenoxymethylpenicillin at 1,000,000 I.U. was added to the treatment twice a day for a period of 10 days, which lasted until the end of hospitalization. Previously administered antibiotics were discontinued. In addition, during hospitalization, the patient was treated intravenously with parenteral hydration (variable values), multi-electrolyte fluid (QD), and Furosemide (BID). The following drugs were administered orally: Spironolactone (QD), Paracetamol (QID), Ibuprofen (to be taken when it was necessary), Clemastine (QD), and a drug containing Magnesia hydroaspartas and Kalii hydroaspartas (to be taken when it was necessary).

2.1.4. Post-Hospital Recommendations

The recommendations included the implementation of home isolation until the full resolution of all clinical symptoms and the performance of control laboratory tests (urinalysis, complete blood count, total protein, CRP, creatine kinase, and transaminase concentration) with outpatient control of the results by the pediatrician. In addition, it was recommended that the patient avoided excessive physical effort and performed daily weight control on an empty stomach, with the implementation of a diet of easily digestible food. A referral was issued for outpatient follow-up visits to nephrology and cardiology outpatient clinics. In the event of recurrent pre-existing clinical symptoms, the child's mother was advised to report again to the pediatric ward. The total time of the patient's stay in the hospital as a result of hospitalization was 14 days.

2.2. *Patient 2*

2.2.1. Patient Information

A 4-year-old boy was admitted to the emergency room of the Department of Pediatrics late in the evening due to dehydration during the course of gastroenteritis one day after patient no. 1. Over the previous three days before admission, the boy had a high and intense fever reaching 40 °C with a mediocre response to antipyretics. He was significantly weakened, vomiting, and passing liquid stools without pathological admixtures. In addition, according to the parent's assessment, diuresis was significantly reduced compared to the previous days. Over the previous two days before hospital admission, a rash was present on the child's skin, which was diagnosed in an outpatient setting as infectious erythema. During the medical interview, the parents denied having previously contracted COVID-19.

2.2.2. Clinical Findings and Diagnostic Assessment

During the time spent in the emergency room, the physical examination showed abnormalities in addition to signs of increased dehydration; significant weakness (the appearance of a very sick child); and fine-spotted rash on the skin of the face (with a Filatov's triangle), chest, abdomen, and genital area; edema on the hands and feet; a raspberry red tongue; and a reddened throat with swollen red tonsils. On the second day of hospitalization, the skin rash became "brushy". Pastia's lines appeared in the groin and elbow folds, and the Filatov triangle became very pronounced.

Blood, urine, and feces samples were taken. The preliminary laboratory tests showed elevated parameters of inflammation and hyponatremia, and significantly elevated activity of transaminases (Table 1). The quantitative test for antibodies on the second day gave a negative result. Due to the characteristic symptoms, a pharyngeal culture for GAS was not ordered. Control laboratory tests, including inflammatory parameters, were performed after 48 and 96 h of hospitalization and at the end of therapy, i.e., on the 10th day of therapy (Table 2).

During hospitalization, three abdominal and retroperitoneal ultrasounds and two lung ultrasounds were performed. The first abdominal examination was performed on the third day of hospitalization, showing a slight amount of interloop fluid in the right iliac fossa and hepatomegaly, which did not change in the control examination performed after 24 h. Another control examination of the abdomen performed on the eighth day of hospitalization showed a significant improvement in the form of a reduction in the amount of interloop fluid. The first ultrasound examination of the lungs performed on the third day of hospitalization showed the presence of fluid in both pleural cavities, hepatosis of the lower lobe of the left lung, and numerous small consolidations within the right lung. The control lung examination carried out on the eighth day of hospitalization showed a regression of inflammatory changes in the lungs.

On the second and ninth days of hospitalization, the patient underwent cardiological consultations. The performed electrocardiographic and echocardiographic examinations showed no significant deviations from the normal state. Additionally, on the second day of hospitalization, an ENT consultation was carried out, which revealed a vivid red throat, reddened tonsils, and swollen deposits on the back of the throat along with purulent discharge. The performed posteroanterior view (PA) + lateral chest X-ray on the ninth day showed lung areas without focal changes and a silhouette of the heart within normal limits.

2.2.3. Therapeutic Interventions and Outcome

Initially, intensive parenteral hydration was used therapeutically. On the day of admission, the patient was treated with Ceftriaxone at a dose of 50/mg/kg/day in intravenous form, which lasted until the eighth day. On that day, the boy had an intense fever reaching 39 °C and was very weak. He had diuresis, but despite the use of parenteral hydration, it was significantly limited. It amounted to 350 mL per 24 h. Persistent peripheral edema and a rapid enlargement of the abdominal circumference were also noticed.

Due to the characteristic features of scarlet fever on the second day of hospitalization, a diagnosis was made in this regard. On that day, Phenoxymethylpenicillin at 1,000,000 I.U. was administered orally twice a day until the end of hospitalization in a dose appropriate to the patient's age, along with a probiotic that had a strain of *Saccharomyces boulardii*. The probiotic was used due to continued diarrhea. The following treatments were administered to the patient intravenously: parenteral hydration (variable values), multi-electrolyte fluid (QD), Furosemide (BID), and Paracetamol (BID). The following drugs were used orally: Spironolactone (BID), Ibuprofen (to be taken when it was necessary), Cetirizine hydrochloride (BID), and inhalations with Budesonide (QD).

2.2.4. Post-Hospital Recommendations

The recommendations included home isolation until complete recovery. Control laboratory tests were also recommended about a week later (urinalysis, aminotransferase concentration, complete blood count, total protein, and CRP), together with a consultation at the pediatric clinic. Avoidance of excessive physical effort, daily weight control on an empty stomach, and a diet of easily digestible food were also recommended. A referral for an outpatient follow-up visit to a nephrology clinic was issued. If pre-existing clinical symptoms recurred, the child's mother was advised to return to the pediatric ward. The total time of the patient's stay in the hospital was 10 days.

2.3. *Comparison of Cases*

Due to the initially severe clinical condition presented in both boys, the possibility of a systemic inflammatory reaction after recovering from COVID-19 was taken into account. Laboratory diagnostics were extended in accordance with the PIMS-TS protocol with a repetition frequency depending on clinical needs. After the introduction of antibiotic therapy, a significant decrease in inflammatory markers and aminotransferase activity was found in both patients. The concentrations of triglycerides were surprisingly high, while cholesterol and total protein levels were significantly lower. Minor disorders of the coagulation system were observed (Table 2). The imaging examinations performed at the Department of Pediatrics showed inflammatory changes in lung ultrasound (consolidations, pleural effusion), as well as significant leaks into the third space in the abdominal cavity.

The unusual similarity between both boys during the clinical course of the disease, as well as the changes in the laboratory and imaging tests, are noteworthy. For logistical reasons, the boys were placed in one patient room during hospitalization. They turned out to be friends from one kindergarten in the same group, where an outbreak of scarlet fever had been diagnosed a few days earlier.

Recognition of the disease as scarlet fever in case no. 2 was considered from the very beginning, while in case no. 1, due to the lack of characteristic symptoms within the first few days of hospitalization, the disease was only recognized after obtaining a throat swab and information from his medical history. After appropriate treatment was implemented, the condition of boy no. 1 improved rapidly (Table 2).

3. Discussion

In Poland, there is an obligation to report infectious diseases, infections, deaths, and biological pathogens to the state sanitary inspectorate. This includes scarlet fever. The epidemiological data prepared by the National Institute of Public Health (NIH)—National Research Institute indicate a significant increase in the number of incidents (per 100,000 inhabitants) of scarlet fever in 2022 (33.09) compared to the previous year (6.94). This is due to the reduced transmission of biological pathogens caused by the SARS-CoV-2 pandemic in 2021, which resulted in restrictions on the movement and attendance of children and young people in kindergartens and schools, as well as reduced access to stationary medical consultations during the pandemic. The highest number of cases in Poland was observed in the first quarter of the year. The statistical data show that 1415 scarlet fevers were diagnosed in Poland in the first half of 2021. This is an incidence rate of 3.71 per 100,000 inhabitants. In the first half of 2022, 5269 cases were already diagnosed, giving an incidence rate of 13.81 per 100,000 inhabitants. On the other hand, the highest number of cases by age falls in the age ranges of 0–4 and 5–9, with a higher incidence among boys. The number of hospitalizations resulting from scarlet fever in the discussed years did not exceed 2.5%, and no deaths caused by this disease were recorded [7,8].

Usually, the course of scarlet fever is mild, and a return to normal activity occurs after two days with the use of appropriate treatment; very rarely is it a reason for hospitalization [2].

In its classic course, scarlet fever remains a fairly simple disease to recognize. The patients described in this paper, however, were difficult cases to diagnose due to symptoms that could be indicative of several other childhood diseases. Patient no. 2 had the characteristic features: a distinctive rash, a Filatov's triangle, a raspberry red tongue, and white coating. Patient no. 1 also had a confluent erythema on his face, and oral examination was limited due to severe inflammation of the gums, tongue, and lips, with significant damage to the mucous membranes.

Both patients gave the impression of "very sick children". Their activity was significantly reduced, and the fever responded poorly to antipyretics. A big problem was the limitation of diuresis, causing peripheral edema of the feet, hands, and sacro-lumbar region. The fluid balance, which was maintained for several days, leveled off only after the use of diuretics. The patients had no record of family history of immunodeficiency or serious bacterial infections. The entire clinical picture gives grounds for considering the existence of a toxic form of *streptococcus pyogenes* infection.

Finally, the throat swab as the main standard enabled the final diagnosis of patient no. 1. The common source of infection, i.e., the kindergarten group and contact with a confirmed case of scarlet fever, left no doubt that it was indeed this disease. After the implementation of a dedicated treatment (phenoxymethyl penicillin), intensive parenteral hydration, diuretic treatment, and use of albumin specimens (in patient 1) with meticulous fluid balance, the boys' clinical condition gradually improved. The patients were discharged in good general condition with recommendations after several days of hospitalization.

The possible impact of surviving a SARS-CoV-2 infection in children remains an open question. Patient no. 1 was infected with the Sars-Cov-2 virus shortly before the mentioned infection, and Patient no. 2 had a negative history. This information was confirmed by a screening test for the presence of antibodies to this virus. Taking into account the location of the Department of Pediatrics (Silesia region), the boys' clinical condition, and the initial test results, PIMS-TS syndrome was suspected. Finally, the patients did not meet the criteria for diagnosis, and the treatment implemented was adequately effective.

Another disease that was initially considered was Epstein–Barr virus (EBV) infection with a severe course (a high temperature, cervical lymphadenopathy, hepatosplenomegaly, and swollen tonsils). Patient no. 1 tested positive in a heterophile antibody screening; however, both boys tested negative for EBV specific antibodies.

The etiology of acute pharyngitis is usually viral. In order not to unnecessarily administer an antibiotic, it is necessary to introduce differential diagnostics, such as pharyngeal cultures for bacteria. The leading agent in this group is *streptococcus pyogenes*. Diagnosis based solely on the clinical image can sometimes be quite difficult. This is because oropharyngeal lesions are not always present in positive cases of infection by GAS. Proper management avoids the development of the problem of antibiotic resistance in patients with GAS [5].

Both the CDC and the Canadian Pediatric Society have established criteria for *Group A Streptococcal* toxic shock syndrome. These patients meet the criteria for probable toxic shock [9,10]. In the literature, cases of toxic shock that are caused by *streptococcus pyogenes* can be found, in which mortality in the pediatric population can be very high, and complications are extremely dangerous [11,12].

Lamagni and colleagues investigated factors that may contribute to the generalization and severity of *S. pyogenes* infection. Based on cases in Greece, a conclusion was drawn about virological factors favoring a severe course of the disease, which may include chickenpox. A patient's current condition should also be confronted with data about vaccinations and past infectious diseases [12–14].

4. Conclusions

Scarlet fever is generally a mild childhood disease, but the possibility of a severe course requiring hospitalization also exists. Therefore, this disease should not be marginalized by other infectious diseases. A diagnosis can be made on the basis of clinical symptoms, but these symptoms are not always clear. Differential diagnosis with other diseases is required. Medical history, which is often very detailed, can be the solution to making a definitive diagnosis and can complement the data collected from the laboratory tests performed.

Author Contributions: Conceptualization K.S.-G., D.K. and K.S.-T.; methodology K.S.-G. and K.S.-T.; formal analysis K.S.-T.; writing—review and editing K.S.-G., D.K. and K.S.-T.; visualization D.K. All authors have read and agreed to the published version of the manuscript.

Funding: This research received no external funding.

Institutional Review Board Statement: This study was conducted in accordance with the Declaration of Helsinki. Ethical review and approval were not required for case studies according to the national regulations in Poland.

Informed Consent Statement: Written informed consent was obtained from the parents of the subjects involved in the study. No personal information that could identify the patients is included.

Data Availability Statement: All relevant data are within the manuscript.

Conflicts of Interest: The authors declare no conflict of interest.

References

1. Carapetis, J.R.; Steer, A.C.; Mulholland, E.K.; Weber, M. The global burden of group A streptococcal diseases. *Lancet Infect. Dis.* **2005**, *5*, 685–694. [CrossRef]
2. Herdman, M.T.; Cordery, R.; Karo, B.; Purba, A.K.; Begum, L.; Lamagni, T.; Kee, C.; Balasegaram, S.; Sriskandan, S. Clinical management and impact of scarlet fever in the modern era: Findings from a cross-sectional study of cases in London, 2018–2019. *BMJ Open* **2021**, *11*, e057772. [CrossRef]
3. Lepoutre, A.; Doloy, A.; Bidet, P.; Leblond, A.; Perrocheau, A.; Bingen, E.; Trieu-Cuot, P.; Bouvet, A.; Poyart, C.; Lévy-Bruhl, D.; et al. Epidemiology of Invasive Streptococcus pyogenes Infections in France in 2007. *J. Clin. Microbiol.* **2011**, *49*, 4094–4100. [CrossRef] [PubMed]
4. Miron, V.D.; Bar, G.; Filimon, C.; Gaidamut, V.A.; Craiu, M. Streptococcal pharyngitis in children: A tertiary pediatric hospital in Bucharest, Romania. *J. Glob. Infect. Dis.* **2021**, *13*, 154. [CrossRef]
5. Miron, V.D.; Craiu, M. "Red throat" or acute pharyngitis—Challenges in real life clinical practice. *Germs* **2021**, *11*, 351–353. [CrossRef] [PubMed]
6. Kennis, M.; Tagawa, A.; Kung, V.M.; Montalbano, G.; Narvaez, I.; Franco-Paredes, C.; Barahona, L.V.; Madinger, N.; Shapiro, L.; Chastain, D.B.; et al. Seasonal variations and risk factors of *Streptococcus pyogenes* infection: A multicenter research network study. *Ther. Adv. Infect. Dis.* **2022**, *9*, 20499361221132101. [CrossRef]
7. Cases of Selected Infectious Diseases in Poland from 1 January to 15 August 2022 and in the Comparable Period of 2021. Available online: http://wwwold.pzh.gov.pl/oldpage/epimeld/2022/INF_22_08A.pdf (accessed on 5 December 2022).
8. Infectious Diseases and Poisonings in Poland in 2021. National Institute of Public Health NIH-National Research Institute. Warsaw; 2022. Available online: http://wwwold.pzh.gov.pl/oldpage/epimeld/2021/Ch_2021.pdf (accessed on 5 December 2022).
9. Centers for Disease Control and Prevention. Available online: https://www.cdc.gov/groupastrep/diseases-hcp/Streptococcal-Toxic-Shock-Syndrome.html (accessed on 10 December 2022).
10. Canadian Paediatric Society. Available online: https://cps.ca/en/documents/position/invasive-group-a-streptococcal-disease (accessed on 10 December 2022).
11. De Carvalho, H.T.; Fioretto, J.R.; Ribeiro, C.F.; Laraia, I.O.; Carpi, M.F. Diagnosis and treatment of streptococcal toxic shock syndrome in the pediatric intensive care unit: Case report. *Rev. Bras. Ter. Intensiv.* **2019**, *31*, 586–591. [CrossRef] [PubMed]
12. Lamagni, T.L.; Neal, S.; Keshishian, C.; Alhaddad, N.; George, R.; Duckworth, G.; Vuopio-Varkila, J.; Efstratiou, A. Severe*Streptococcus pyogenes*Infections, United Kingdom, 2003–2004. *Emerg. Infect. Dis.* **2008**, *14*, 202–209. [CrossRef] [PubMed]
13. Watts, V.; Balasegaram, S.; Brown, C.S.; Mathew, S.; Mearkle, R.; Ready, D.; Saliba, V.; Lamagni, T. Increased Risk for Invasive Group A*Streptococcus*Disease for Household Contacts of Scarlet Fever Cases, England, 2011–2016. *Emerg. Infect. Dis.* **2019**, *25*, 529–537. [CrossRef] [PubMed]
14. Luca-Harari, B.; Darenberg, J.; Neal, S.; Siljander, T.; Strakova, L.; Tanna, A.; Creti, R.; Ekelund, K.; Koliou, M.; Tassios, P.T.; et al. Clinical and Microbiological Characteristics of Severe *Streptococcus pyogenes* Disease in Europe. *J. Clin. Microbiol.* **2009**, *47*, 1155–1165. [CrossRef] [PubMed]

children

MDPI

Case Report

Spontaneous Pneumomediastinum in Children with Viral Infections: Report of Three Cases Related to Rhinovirus or Respiratory Syncytial Virus Infection

Johanna L. Leinert [1,2], Alba Perez Ortiz [2] and Neysan Rafat [2,*]

1 University Children's Hospital, Medical Faculty Mannheim, Heidelberg University, 68167 Mannheim, Germany; johanna.leinert@umm.de

2 Department of Neonatology, Medical Faculty Mannheim, Heidelberg University, 68167 Mannheim, Germany; alba.perez-ortiz@umm.de

* Correspondence: neysan.rafat@umm.de

Abstract: Background: Spontaneous pneumomediastinum (SP) is generally a benign condition which can have various etiologies. Data on SP related to respiratory viral infections in children are rare and there are currently no official guidelines or consistent treatment recommendations for these patients. Aim: To discuss treatment options considering the recommendations for SP with different etiologies. Methods: We report three cases of SP, which were related to rhinovirus or respiratory syncytial virus (RSV) infection. Results: All three patients presented with typical symptoms of a respiratory tract infection and required oxygen supplementation during the hospital stay. All children benefited from a conservative, supportive therapy, and bed rest, and could be discharged after seven days or less without remaining symptoms. Conclusion: Surveillance and monitoring might be reasonable to detect and treat potential complications in children with SP due to viral infections, as one child developed an increasing pneumothorax, which had to be treated with a thoracic drainage.

Keywords: pneumomediastinum; children; viral infection; rhinovirus infection

1. Introduction

A pneumomediastinum is generally defined as the presence of interstitial air in the mediastinum. A spontaneous pneumomediastinum (SP) is caused by an increased pressure in the airways in comparison to the surrounding tissue, leading to a spread of air into the mediastinum without any external cause, such as trauma or surgery. In this incidence, air is often also pressed into the subcutaneous tissue or the pleural space, which is why an SP is often accompanied with subcutaneous emphysema and pneumothoraces [1]. In most cases, an SP presents with mild symptoms of chest and neck pain, sore throat, or dyspnea [2]. In children, SPs occur most commonly in asthma exacerbation or after a Valsalva maneuver such as vomiting or coughing [3–5]. Other triggering factors can be bronchospasms or foreign body ingestions. Only 13% to 20% of SPs have been described as occurring related to viral infections [4,5]. Recently they have also been described for patients with COVID-19 infections [6–8].

SPs related to respiratory viral infections in children are rare and only a few case reports are published [9,10]. Studies focusing on SPs due to respiratory viral infections are not available. Accordingly, data regarding the clinical course in these patients is rare, and there are currently no official guidelines or consistent treatment recommendations for those patients.

In this work, we report three cases of SP, which were related to rhinovirus or respiratory syncytial virus (RSV) infection in children, and discuss treatment options for these patients, considering the recommendations for SPs with different etiologies.

2. Case Reports

2.1. Case 1

Patient 1 was a three-year-old girl presenting with fever and cough for two days as well as tachydyspnea and neck swelling. In the clinical examination subcutaneous emphysema was detected above the clavicles and bilateral rhonchus was auscultated. Accordingly, a chest X-ray was performed, which showed a pneumomediastinum and a large subcutaneous emphysema (Figure 1). A polymerase chain reaction (PCR) of the nasal secretions obtained in our emergency unit was positive for RSV. High C-reactive protein (CRP) levels (108 mg/L, normal range 0–5 mg/L) led to the assumption of bacterial superinfection, which led to a treatment with ampicillin (100 mg per kg body weight per day, divided in three doses) for seven days. Oxygen supplementation was necessary to keep the saturation between 88% and 92%. Afterwards, oxygen supplementation could be stopped as the saturation was normal. Additionally, she received supportive intravenous fluid, and bed rest was prescribed. She recovered and was discharged after seven days.

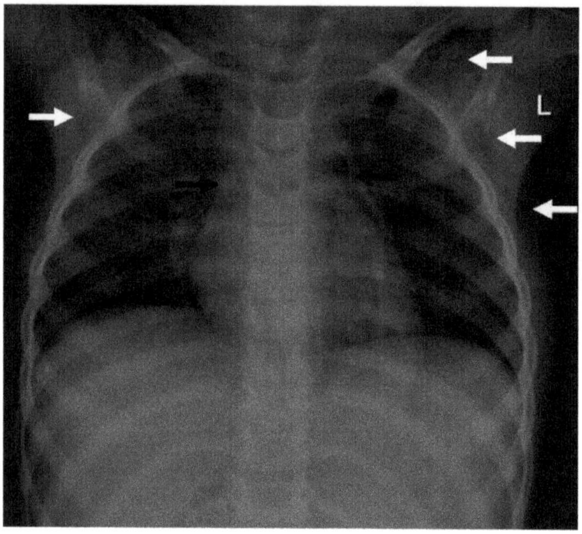

Figure 1. Imaging findings in patient 1. Chest X-ray showing a pneumomediastinum (black arrows) and a subcutaneous emphysema, more pronounced on the left site (white arrows).

2.2. Case 2

Patient 2 was a three-year-old girl with a history of three days of fever, obstructive bronchitis, and dyspnea, as well as a cough with sputum. On physical examination she presented with bilateral wheezing, rattling noises, and palpable subcutaneous emphysema. Multiplex PCR of the nasopharyngeal aspirate revealed an acute rhinovirus infection. In addition, this patient was treated with antibiotics due to bacterial superinfection (also suspected because of elevated CRP levels (99 mg/L) and received intravenous fluids (1.2 L of saline per day (85 mL/kg/day)). Therapy with the broad-spectrum antibiotic agent ceftriaxone (75 mg per kg body weight per day) had already been started by the referring hospital. To treat the obstructive bronchitis, she received inhalation treatment with salbutamol and corticosteroids. She required oxygen supplementation via nasal canula to maintain an oxygen saturation > 94%. Chest radiograph showed a pneumomediastinum in combination with pneumothorax and subcutaneous emphysema (Figure 2A). Due to deterioration of symptoms a follow-up X-ray was performed and indicated an increase in the pneumothorax and pneumomediastinum. A subsequent computed tomography (CT) of the thorax showed the increasing pneumomediastinum and pneumothorax, as well as bilateral atelectases (Figure 2B,C). Because of pulmonary deterioration with increasing dyspnea, a thoracic drainage was applied to treat the pneumothorax, which led to improvement within the next days. The patient recovered, the drainage could be removed after three days, and she was discharged after seven days.

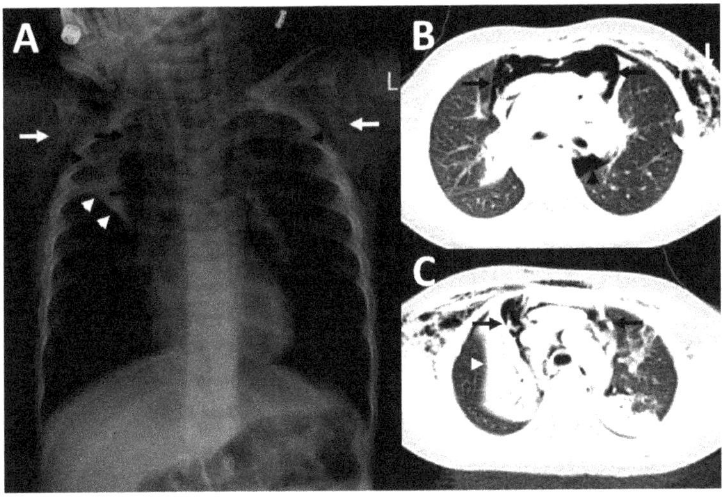

Figure 2. Imaging findings in patient 2. In the chest x-ray (**A**), as well as in CT-imaging (**B**,**C**) bilateral subcutaneous emphysema (white arrows) and a pneumomediastinum (black arrows) with a Spinnaker sail (angel wing) sign ((**A**), thymus lobes marked with black arrowheads) was detected. In addition, there were atelectases (white arrowheads), predominantly of the right upper lobe, as well as a pneumothorax (black arrowhead in (**B**)).

2.3. Case 3

Patient 3 was a six-and-a-half-year-old girl who was admitted to our hospital with dyspnea and epigastric and chest pain after a history of a respiratory infection during the days before. Because of inspiratory and expiratory stridor, inhalation with bronchodilators was established and oxygen supplementation was started. In the clinical examination, a massive subcutaneous emphysema of the neck and chest was observed. Blood tests detected elevated infection markers (leukocytes of 15.4/nL (normal range 4.7–10.3/nL) and CRP of 58 mg/L). Therefore, we suspected bacterial superinfection and started empiric antibiotic treatment with ampicillin (for dosage, see case 1). Multiplex PCR of the nasal secretion was positive for rhinovirus. An X-ray was performed, showing a pneumomediastinum and pneumothorax as well as a subcutaneous emphysema (Figure 3). Because of suspected pneumopericardium in the chest X-ray and due to aggravation of the patient's symptoms, an additional chest CT was performed. The CT ruled out a pneumopericardium and confirmed the pneumomediastinum and pneumothorax, and additionally showed pneumorrhachis (presence of air in the spinal epidural space). We carefully observed the patient, prescribed bed rest, and performed supportive treatment with oxygen therapy and intravenous fluid. The patient improved within the next few days and an X-ray before discharge showed an improvement of the initial findings. A few days later the symptoms completely resolved, and the patient was discharged after six days.

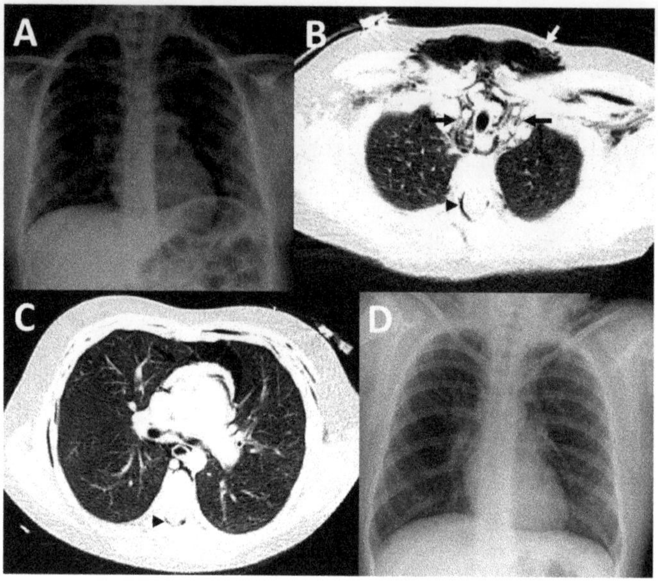

Figure 3. Imaging findings in patient 3. In the initial chest X-ray, pneumopericardium was suspected (**A**). Therefore, a CT was performed (**B**,**C**) which showed a pneumomediastinum (black arrows), accompanied by a large subcutaneous emphysema (white arrow) and epidural pneumatosis (black arrowhead), but no pneumopericardium. A chest X-ray (**D**) which was acquired at discharge showed substantial improvement of the previously mentioned findings.

3. Discussion

In this report, we investigated three cases of children with SP caused by viral infections of the airways who could be effectively managed with supportive therapy, rest, and monitoring.

RSV and rhinovirus are two of the most common pathogens causing viral respiratory infections in children and are often seen in winter and beginning of spring [11]. Children under the age of two years, especially prematurely born toddlers, and those with chronic illnesses, such as immunodeficiencies or broncho-pulmonary disease, are often hospitalized with RSV [11]. The coincidence of RSV infection and SP has only been described in two other case reports before, and only one case of coincident rhinovirus infection and SP has been described [9,10]. The typical symptoms of these infections, dyspnea and coughing, which were present in all of our patients, can lead to an increased intrathoracic pressure, resulting in alveolar rupture, leading to SP.

In children presenting with dyspnea, chest pain, or subcutaneous emphysema, a chest X-ray may be indicated, which normally leads to the diagnosis of SP, if present. In unclear cases or suspected complications, such as pneumopericardium and tension pneumothorax or to exclude an esophageal rupture, a CT scan can be performed, as was the case with patients 2 and 3 of our report. In patient 3, we also observed a pneumorrhachis, which may appear to be a serious complication. However, previous studies showed that pneumorrhachis is self-limiting and does not require specific treatment in the vast majority of cases [12].

All three of our patients received supportive therapy with oxygen via nasal cannula and intravenous fluids which led to a substantial improvement of their symptoms. In all cases, blood tests showed increased inflammatory markers (leucocytes and CRP), which lead to the suspicion of bacterial superinfection. Therefore, all children received empiric intravenous antibiotic treatment. Only patient 2 needed additional invasive treatment in terms of a thoracic drainage to treat an enlarging pneumothorax which caused increasing dyspnea.

There are currently no guidelines and only a few treatment recommendations for children with SP. This might contribute to the fact that SP is often overinvestigated and overtreated [9,12,13]. Our cases suggest that SP in children with viral infections can be effectively treated with the above-mentioned supportive therapies.

A few larger studies investigated children with SP; however, in these studies the underlying cause for SP was manifold and their conclusions and recommendations were not restricted to or focused on viral infections [4,5,14]. In addition, two review articles were published, summarizing the diagnosis and management of children with SP; however, these also did not specifically address the etiology of the disease [1,15]. These studies and reviews recommend a conservative, non-invasive treatment for pediatric patients with SP, which is in line with our management. Noorbakhsh et al. and Fitzwater et al., who studied 183 and 96 children, respectively, concluded that short-term observation of a child with SP with mild symptoms in the emergency department might be sufficient [4,5]. In the study by Fitzwater et al., in most cases children were admitted to the hospital and some also to the ICU, although none of them had progression or were intubated [4]. We think that hospitalization for children suffering from SP secondary to viral infections might be reasonable to enable rest and monitoring, and especially to enable treatment and detection of imminent or already present complications.

In conclusion, SP related to viral infections appears to be a benign condition. Supportive treatment and rest are effective therapies for SP. Surveillance and monitoring might be reasonable to detect and treat potential complications.

Author Contributions: Conceptualization, methodology, and original draft preparation: J.L.L. and N.R. Writing, review, and editing: J.L.L., A.P.O. and N.R. All authors have read and agreed to the published version of the manuscript.

Funding: This research received no external funding.

Institutional Review Board Statement: The study was conducted in accordance with the Declaration of Helsinki. Ethical review and approval were not required for case studies according to the national regulations.

Informed Consent Statement: Written informed consent was obtained from the parents of the subjects involved in the study.

Data Availability Statement: All relevant data are within the manuscript.

Conflicts of Interest: The authors declare no conflict of interest.

References

1. Bullaro, F.M.; Bartoletti, S.C. Spontaneous pneumomediastinum in children: A literature review. *Pediatr. Emerg. Care* **2007**, *23*, 28–30. [CrossRef] [PubMed]
2. Sahni, S.; Verma, S.; Grullon, J.; Esquire, A.; Patel, P.; Talwar, A. Spontaneous pneumomediastinum: Time for consensus. *N. Am. J. Med. Sci.* **2013**, *5*, 460–464. [PubMed]
3. Chalumeau, M.; Le Clainche, L.; Sayeg, N.; Sannier, N.; Michel, J.L.; Marianowski, R.; Jouvet, P.; Scheinmann, P.; de Blic, J. Spontaneous pneumomediastinum in children. *Pediatr. Pulmonol.* **2001**, *31*, 67–75. [CrossRef]
4. Fitzwater, J.W.; Silva, N.N.; Knight, C.G.; Malvezzi, L.; Ramos-Irizarry, C.; Burnweit, C.A. Management of spontaneous pneumomediastinum in children. *J. Pediatr. Surg.* **2015**, *50*, 983–986. [CrossRef] [PubMed]
5. Noorbakhsh, K.A.; Williams, A.E.; Langham, J.J.W.; Wu, L.; Krafty, R.T.; Furtado, A.D.; Zuckerbraun, N.S.; Manole, M.D. Management and Outcomes of Spontaneous Pneumomediastinum in Children. *Pediatr. Emerg. Care* **2019**, *37*, e1051–e1056. [CrossRef] [PubMed]
6. Iuorio, A.; Nagar, F.; Attianese, L.; Grasso, A.; Torretta, G.; Fusco, P.; Ferrara, M.; Ferraro, F. Spontaneous Pneumomediastinum and Pneumothorax in Nonintubated COVID-19 Patients: A Multicenter Case Series. *Am. J. Case Rep.* **2021**, *22*, e933405. [CrossRef] [PubMed]
7. Baratella, E.; Bussani, R.; Zanconati, F.; Marrocchio, C.; Fabiola, G.; Braga, L.; Maiocchi, S.; Berlot, G.; Volpe, M.C.; Moro, E.; et al. Radiological-pathological signatures of patients with COVID-19-related pneumomediastinum: Is there a role for the Sonic hedgehog and Wnt5a pathways? *ERJ Open Res.* **2021**, *7*, 00346-2021. [CrossRef] [PubMed]
8. Jagosz, M.; Guzik, W.; Moczala, L.; Rydel, M.; Misiolek, H.; Bialka, S. Young convalescent COVID-19 pneumonia with extensive pneumomediastinum emphysema: Case report. *Clin. Case Rep.* **2022**, *10*, e05543. [CrossRef] [PubMed]

9. Emiralioglu, N.; Ozcan, H.N.; Oguz, B.; Yalcin, E.; Dogru, D.; Ozcelik, U.; Kiper, N. Pneumomediastinum, pneumorrhachis and subcutaneous emphysema associated with viral infections: Report of three cases. *Pediatr. Int.* **2015**, *57*, 1038–1040. [CrossRef]
10. Dehmel, M.; Demirakca, S.; Jordan, A.; Dahlheim, M.; Diehm, T.; Schroten, H.; Tenenbaum, T. Pneumomediastinum and subcutaneus emphysema—An uncommon presentation of respiratory-syncytial virus infection in an infant. *Klin Padiatr.* **2013**, *225*, 230–231. [CrossRef]
11. Manoha, C.; Espinosa, S.; Aho, S.L.; Huet, F.; Pothier, P. Epidemiological and clinical features of hMPV, RSV and RVs infections in young children. *J. Clin. Virol.* **2007**, *38*, 221–226. [CrossRef] [PubMed]
12. Oertel, M.F.; Korinth, M.C.; Reinges, M.H.; Krings, T.; Terbeck, S.; Gilsbach, J.M. Pathogenesis, diagnosis and management of pneumorrhachis. *Eur. Spine J.* **2006**, *15* (Suppl. 5), 636–643. [CrossRef] [PubMed]
13. Caceres, M.; Ali, S.Z.; Braud, R.; Weiman, D.; Garrett, H.E., Jr. Spontaneous pneumomediastinum: A comparative study and review of the literature. *Ann. Thorac. Surg.* **2008**, *86*, 962–966. [CrossRef] [PubMed]
14. Abbas, P.I.; Akinkuotu, A.C.; Peterson, M.L.; Mazziotti, M.V. Spontaneous pneumomediastinum in the pediatric patient. *Am. J. Surg.* **2015**, *210*, 1031–1035, discussion 1035–1036. [CrossRef] [PubMed]
15. Gasser, C.R.; Pellaton, R.; Rochat, C.P. Pediatric Spontaneous Pneumomediastinum: Narrative Literature Review. *Pediatr. Emerg. Care* **2017**, *33*, 370–374. [CrossRef] [PubMed]

children MDPI

Article

Impact of the First COVID Lockdown on Accident- and Injury-Related Pediatric Intensive Care Admissions in Germany—A Multicenter Study

Nora Bruns [1,*], Lea Y. Willemsen [1], Katharina Holtkamp [1], Oliver Kamp [2], Marcel Dudda [2], Bernd Kowall [3], Andreas Stang [3], Florian Hey [4], Judith Blankenburg [5], Hemmen Sabir [6], Frank Eifinger [7], Hans Fuchs [8], Roland Haase [9], Clemens Andrée [10], Michael Heldmann [11], Jenny Potratz [12], Daniel Kurz [13], Anja Schumann [14], Merle Müller-Knapp [15], Nadine Mand [16], Claus Doerfel [17], Peter Dahlem [18], Tobias Rothoeft [19], Manuel Ohlert [20], Katrin Silkenbäumer [21], Frank Dohle [22], Fithri Indraswari [23], Frank Niemann [24], Peter Jahn [25], Michael Merker [26], Nicole Braun [27], Francisco Brevis Nunez [28], Matthias Engler [29], Konrad Heimann [30], Gerhard K. Wolf [31], Dominik Wulf [32], Saskia Hankel [33], Holger Freymann [34], Nicolas Allgaier [35], Felix Knirsch [36], Martin Dercks [37], Julia Reinhard [38], Marc Hoppenz [39], Ursula Felderhoff-Müser [1] and Christian Dohna-Schwake [1]

1 Department of Pediatrics I, Pediatric Intensive Care Medicine, University Medicine Essen, University of Duisburg-Essen, 45147 Essen, Germany; lea.willemsen@stud.uni-due.de (L.Y.W.); katharina.holtkamp@uk-essen.de (K.H.); ursula.felderhoff@uk-essen.de (U.F.-M.); christian.dohna-schwake@uk-essen.de (C.D.-S.)
2 Department of Trauma, Hand and Reconstructive Surgery, University Medicine Essen, University of Duisburg-Essen, 45147 Essen, Germany; oliver.kamp@uk-essen.de (O.K.); marcel.dudda@uk-essen.de (M.D.)
3 Institute of Medical Informatics, Biometry and Epidemiology, University Medicine Essen, University of Duisburg-Essen, 45147 Essen, Germany; bernd.kowall@uk-essen.de (B.K.); imibe.dir@uk-essen.de (A.S.)
4 Pediatric Clinic and Pediatric Polyclinic at the Dr. von Haunersches Children's Hospital, Interdisciplinary Pediatric Intensive Care Unit—Pediatric Emergency Medicine, LMU Munich, 80337 Munich, Germany; florian.hey@med.uni-muenchen.de
5 Department of Pediatrics, Pediatric Intensive Care Medicine, University Hospital Dresden, University of Technology Dresden, 01307 Dresden, Germany; judith.blankenburg@uniklinikum-dresden.de
6 Department of Pediatrics, Neonatology and Pediatric Intensive Care Medicine, University Hospital Bonn, University of Bonn, 53127 Bonn, Germany; hemmen.sabir@ukbonn.de
7 Department of Pediatrics, Pediatric Intensive Care Medicine, University Hospital Cologne, University of Cologne, 50937 Cologne, Germany; frank.eifinger1@uk-koeln.de
8 Department of Pediatrics, Pediatric Intensive Care Medicine, University Hospital Freiburg, University of Freiburg, 79106 Freiburg, Germany; hans.fuchs@uniklinik-freiburg.de
9 Department of Pediatrics, Neonatology and Pediatric Intensive Care Medicine, University Hospital Halle, University of Halle, 06132 Halle, Germany; roland.haase@uk-halle.de
10 Department of Pediatrics, Pediatric Intensive Care Medicine, Helios Hospital Krefeld, 47805 Krefeld, Germany; clemens.andree@helios-gesundheit.de
11 Department of Pediatrics, Pediatric Intensive Care Medicine, Helios University Hospital Wuppertal, 42283 Wuppertal, Germany; michael.heldmann@helios-gesundheit.de
12 Department of Pediatrics, Pediatric Intensive Care Medicine, University Hospital, 48149 Münster, Germany; jenny.potratz@ukmuenster.de
13 Department of Pediatrics 3, Pediatric Cardiology, Pediatric Intensive Care Medicine, Olgahospital Stuttgart, 70174 Stuttgart, Germany; d.kurz@klinikum-stuttgart.de
14 Department of Pediatrics, Pediatric Intensive Care Medicine, Schwarzwald-Baar Hospital Villingen-Schwenningen, 78052 Villingen-Schwenningen, Germany; anja.schumann@sbk-vs.de
15 Department of Pediatrics, Pediatric Intensive Care Medicine, University Hospital, University of Rostock, 18057 Rostock, Germany; merle.muellerknapp@gmail.com
16 Department of Pediatrics, Pediatric Intensive Care Medicine, University Hospital, Philipps University of Marburg, 35043 Marburg, Germany; mandn@staff.uni-marburg.de
17 Department of Pediatrics, Pediatric Intensive Care Medicine, University Hospital Jena, University of Jena, 07747 Jena, Germany; claus.doerfel@med.uni-jena.de
18 Department of Pediatrics, Pediatric Intensive Care Medicine, Hospital Coburg, 96450 Coburg, Germany; peter.dahlem@regiomed-kliniken.de
19 Department of Pediatrics, Pediatric Intensive Care Medicine, Catholic Hospital Bochum, Ruhr-University of Bochum, 44791 Bochum, Germany; tobias.rothoeft@klinikum-bochum.de

[20] Department of Pediatrics, Pediatric Intensive Care Medicine, Community Hospital Koblenz, 56068 Koblenz, Germany; manuel.ohlert@gk.de
[21] Department of Pediatrics, Pediatric Intensive Care Medicine, Protestant Hospital Bethel, University of Bielefeld, 33615 Bielefeld, Germany; katrin.silkenbaeumer@evkb.de
[22] Department of Pediatrics, Pediatric Intensive Care Medicine, St. Vinzenz Hospital Paderborn, 33098 Paderborn, Germany; f.dohle@vincenz.de
[23] Department of Pediatrics, Pediatric Intensive Care Medicine, Hospital Fulda, 36043 Fulda, Germany; fithri.indraswari@klinikum-fulda.de
[24] Department of Pediatrics, Pediatric Intensive Care Medicine, Bergmannsheil and Pediatric Hospital Buer, 45894 Gelsenkirchen, Germany; frank.niemann@kjkge.de
[25] Department of Pediatrics, Pediatric Intensive Care Medicine, Hospital Leverkusen GmbH, 51375 Leverkusen, Germany; peter.jahn@klinikum-lev.de
[26] Department for Children and Adolescents, Division for Stem Cell Transplantation, Immunology and Intensive Care Medicine, University Hospital Frankfurt, Goethe University, 60596 Frankfurt am Main, Germany; michael.merker@kgu.de
[27] Department of Surgery III, Pediatric Surgery, Ernst von Bergmann Hospital of Potsdam, 14467 Potsdam, Germany; nicole.braun@klinikumevb.de
[28] Department of Pediatrics, Pediatric Intensive Care Medicine, Sana Hospitals Duisburg, 47055 Duisburg, Germany; francisco.brevis@sana.de
[29] Department of Pediatrics, Pediatric Intensive Care Medicine, Sana Hospital Offenbach, 63069 Offenbach, Germany; matthias.engler@sana.de
[30] Department of Pediatrics, Pediatric Intensive Care Medicine, University Hospital Aachen, RWTH Aachen University, 52074 Aachen, Germany; kheimann@ukaachen.de
[31] Department of Pediatrics, Pediatric Intensive Care Medicine, Hospital of Traunstein, Southeast Bavaria Hospitals, 83278 Traunstein, Germany; gerhard.wolf@kliniken-sob.de
[32] Department of Pediatrics, Pediatric Intensive Care Medicine, University Hospital Düsseldorf, Heinrich Heine University of Düsseldorf, 40225 Düsseldorf, Germany; dominik.wulf@med.uni-duesseldorf.de
[33] Department of Pediatrics, Pediatric Surgery and Pediatric Intensive Care Medicine, Hospital of Dortmund, 44137 Dortmund, Germany; saskia.hankel@klinikumdo.de
[34] Department of Pediatrics, Pediatric Intensive Care Medicine, Florence Nightingale Hospital, 40489 Düsseldorf, Germany; freymann@kaiserswerther-diakonie.de
[35] Department of Pediatrics, Pediatric Intensive Care Medicine, University Hospital Augsburg, University of Augsburg, 86156 Augsburg, Germany; n.allgaier@gmx.de
[36] Department of Pediatrics, Pediatric Intensive Care Medicine, Sana Hospital Remscheid, 42859 Remscheid, Germany; felix.knirsch@sana.de
[37] Department of Pediatrics, Pediatric Intensive Care Medicine, Clemenshospital Münster, 48153 Münster, Germany; m.dercks@alexianer.de
[38] Department of Pediatrics, Pediatric Intensive Care Medicine, Hospital Mittelbaden, 76532 Baden-Baden, Germany; j.reinhard@klinikum-mittelbaden.de
[39] Department of Pediatrics, Pediatric Intensive Care Medicine, Cologne Hospitals, Children's Hospital Amsterdamer Str., 50735 Cologne, Germany; hoppenzm@kliniken-koeln.de
* Correspondence: nora.bruns@uk-essen.de

Abstract: Children's and adolescents' lives drastically changed during COVID lockdowns worldwide. To compare accident- and injury-related admissions to pediatric intensive care units (PICU) during the first German COVID lockdown with previous years, we conducted a retrospective multicenter study among 37 PICUs (21.5% of German PICU capacities). A total of 1444 admissions after accidents or injuries during the first lockdown period and matched periods of 2017–2019 were reported and standardized morbidity ratios (SMR) were calculated. Total PICU admissions due to accidents/injuries declined from an average of 366 to 346 (SMR 0.95 (CI 0.85–1.05)). Admissions with trauma increased from 196 to 212 (1.07 (0.93–1.23). Traffic accidents and school/kindergarten accidents decreased (0.77 (0.57–1.02 and 0.26 (0.05–0.75)), whereas household and leisure accidents increased (1.33 (1.06–1.66) and 1.34 (1.06–1.67)). Less neurosurgeries and more visceral surgeries were performed (0.69 (0.38–1.16) and 2.09 (1.19–3.39)). Non-accidental non-suicidal injuries declined (0.73 (0.42–1.17)). Suicide attempts increased in adolescent boys (1.38 (0.51–3.02)), but decreased in adolescent girls (0.56 (0.32–0.79)). In summary, changed trauma mechanisms entailed different surgeries compared to previous years. We found no evidence for an increase in child abuse cases requiring intensive care. The increase in suicide attempts among boys demands investigation.

Keywords: accident; trauma; injury; lockdown; pediatric intensive care; COVID

1. Introduction

By the beginning of March 2020, the spread of the new corona virus SARS-CoV had reached most parts of Europe, including Germany. To prevent an uncontrolled transmission of the virus, the German state and federal governments announced drastic restrictions to public and private life. The lockdown came into effect on 16 March and restrained many of children's daily activities. This first lockdown to control the pandemic lasted until the end of May 2020, when restrictions were gradually relaxed.

Several authors have reported drastic declines in pediatric emergency department visits, which were mainly driven by declines in infectious diseases [1–3]. In the Netherlands and New Zealand, less children presented to emergency departments with trauma [4,5]. The lockdown with restrictions to public and private life posed completely new and unknown challenges for families in Germany. Parents had to work at home and simultaneously care for their children, which led to psychosocial stress [6,7]. High rates of clinical anxiety and depression among parents have been reported from the United States during this time [1]. Across countries, there was major public concern that the lockdown restrictions would lead to an increase in unrecognized child abuse due to lack of social control by schools and kindergartens.

The aim of this study was to examine changes in accident- and injury-related admissions to pediatric intensive care units (PICU) during the German COVID lockdown compared to corresponding calendar periods of previous years. To address this issue, we conducted a retrospective observational multi-center study among 37 pediatric intensive care units (PICU) across the country.

2. Methods

2.1. Study Design and Recruitment

The study was designed as a retrospective observational multicenter analysis. Members of an informal mailing list of the German Society of Neonatal and Pediatric Intensive Care (GNPI) were inquired via email to participate in the study. Additionally, German children's hospitals with intensive care units were identified via the homepage of German Society for Pediatrics (Deutsche Gesellschaft für Kinder- und Jugendmedizin). Inquiries for participation in the study were sent out to representatives via email twice between September of 2020 and February of 2021.

2.2. Eligibility and Identification of Cases

Patients < 18 years of age admitted to a German pediatric intensive care unit due to accidents or injuries were eligible. Patients were admitted to the pediatric intensive care unit if they had or were at risk for severe acute decompensation, neurologic deterioration, life-threatening organ dysfunction, hemodynamic instability, or required invasive or continuous monitoring due to the severity of their condition. The evaluation of the clinical condition and decision for PICU admission was at the discretion of the attending physician/hospital. The observation period was the first German lockdown (16 March to 31 May of 2020), the corresponding calendar periods of the years 2017–2019 served as reference period. Eligible diagnoses were S00–S99 and T00–T78 according to the German modification of the ICD system (ICD-10-GM). S codes apply for trauma diagnoses and T codes apply for other types of injuries or damage from external sources. Eligible patients were identified via local hospitals' medical controlling services.

2.3. German Lockdown

The German lockdown came in to effect on 16 March 2020 with school and daycare closures. Recreational facilities including playgrounds were closed and people were urged to reduce their contacts and stay at home. Group gatherings were prohibited. Performing individual sports outside or leaving the house was not prohibited or restricted to a specific distance from home or to a specific length of time. Compared to other European countries such as France, Italy, Spain, and the United Kingdom (UK), the German lockdown was less strict and relied on voluntary participation of the population. Unlike in other countries, restructuring of the health care system was not applied to pediatric departments and pediatric intensive care units, which remained fully functional during the lockdown. From the beginning of May, the lockdown measures were gradually relaxed until 31 May 2020.

2.4. Data Acquisition

Anonymized clinical data were extracted from discharge summaries. Data were entered online into a questionnaire hosted at Microsoft Office Forms 365 for institutional users by the participating centers themselves. Alternatively, anonymized discharge letters were mailed or emailed to the principal study site (Department of Pediatrics I, University Medicine Essen) and entered by local staff (LW and KH) (Figure 1). After the completion of data collection, the raw data were downloaded as a Microsoft Office Excel file and imported into SAS Enterprise Guide 8.4 for statistical analyses.

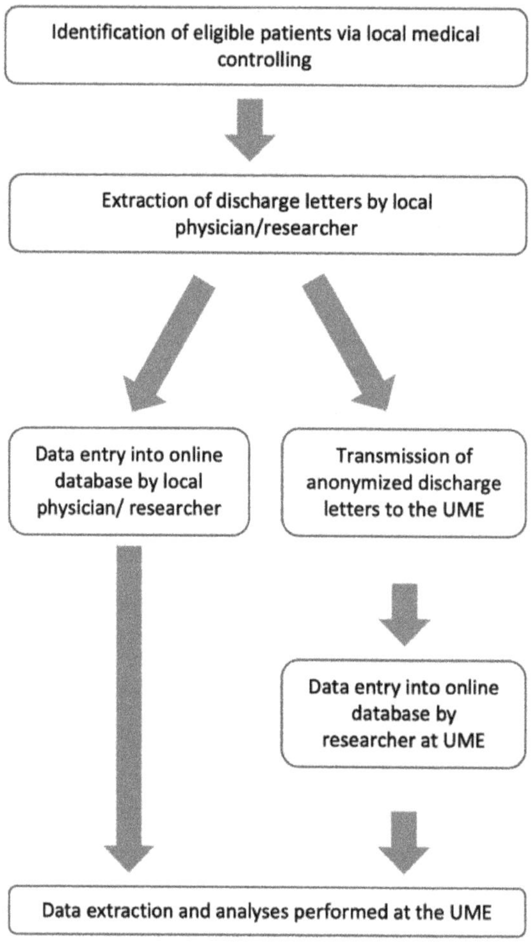

Figure 1. Data flow between participating centers. UME, University Medicine Essen.

To determine the percentage of PICU capacities represented by the participating centers, we accessed the DIVI registry of intensive care beds (German Interdisciplinary Association of Intensive Care and Emergency Medicine, Deutsche interdisziplinäre Vereinigung für Intensiv- und Notfallmedizin) and extracted the total number of PICUs, PICU beds in Germany and the number of beds provided by the participating centers in this study. Some children's hospitals do not report pediatric and neonatal intensive care capacities separately in the DIVI registry. These capacities were ignored for the calculation of the percentage, since we assumed that this is information is missing completely at random.

2.5. Statistical Analyses

Continuous variables are presented as median with interquartile range (IQR) and mean with 95% confidence intervals (CI). For discrete variables, absolute and relative frequencies are given. Standardized morbidity ratios (SMR) for the lockdown period were calculated, adjusting for age and sex. The years from 2017 to 2019 served as reference period to calculate the expected number of cases for 2020. The observed number of cases in 2020 was then divided by the expected number of cases. An SMR > 1 indicates an increase in cases, an SMR < 1 a decrease. We calculated exact 95% CIs if the number of observed events in the lockdown period was <15 and employed the Poisson approximation to calculate CIs in case of ≥15 events [8]. Additionally, *p*-values were calculated for all SMRs.

Age groups for calculation of SMRs were defined as 0–1 years, 2–5 years, 6–11 years, and 12–17 years. Three patients with diverse gender, all from the reference period, were excluded from SMR calculations since no patient with diverse gender was admitted during the observation period.

SAS Enterprise Guide 8.4 (SAS Institute Inc., Cary, NC, USA) was used to perform statistical analyses and produce figures. SISA software [9] was used to calculate exact and Poisson CIs for SMRs.

2.6. Ethics Approval

The study was approved by the ethics committee of the Medical Faculty of the University of Duisburg-Essen (20-9560-BO). Local ethics committees of the participating centers additionally approved of the study if required by local legislation. Data entry and storage in Microsoft Office Forms is in line with the General Data Protection Regulation of the European Union (Regulation (EU) 2016/679).

3. Results

We recruited 37 (23.3%) of 159 German PICUs including 18 University Hospitals. The locations of the hospitals are presented in Figure 2. Of 801 PICU beds listed in the DIVI registry, the participating centers accounted for 172, thereby comprising 21.5% of the German pediatric intensive care capacities. A total of 1483 cases were reported. Thirty-one cases did not fulfill the inclusion criteria, and eight cases with T diagnoses were excluded from analysis since they were not accidents or injuries. This may happen due to the fact that some subcategories of the ICD codes T75, T76, and T78 include non-injury diagnoses. The remaining 1444 cases were analyzed. The median number of reported cases per hospital was 52 (interquartile range 19–118). Clinical details of the included patients are provided in Table 1 and Figure 3.

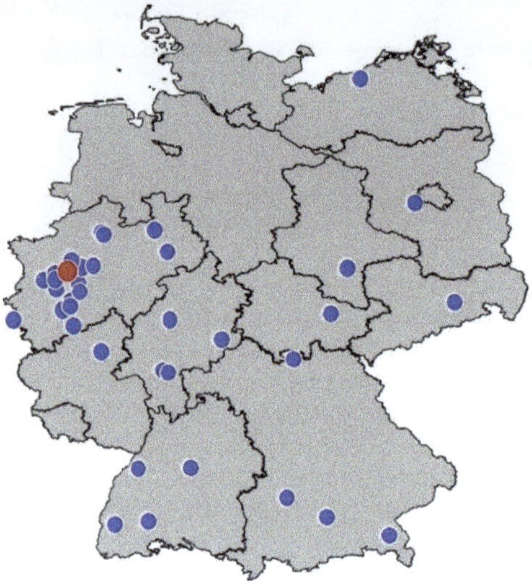

Figure 2. Localization of the participating PICUs. Each circle represents one center. The main study center in Essen (red) is located in the cluster in North Rhine-Westphalia, where 21.6% of the German population live.

Table 1. Patient characteristics.

	Overall *n* (%)	Reference Period (2017–2019) *n* (%)	2020 *n* (%)
Admissions (*n*)	1444	1098	346
Admissions < 1 year of age [*n* (%)]	121 (8.4%)	91 (8.3%)	30 (8.7%)
Age [median (IQR)	6.5 (2–13)	7 (2–14)	6 (2–12)
mean (95% CI)]	7.5 (7.2–7.8)	7.6 (7.3–8.0)	7.3 (6.7–7.8)
Male [*n* (%)]	787 (54.5%)	588 (53.6%)	199 (57.5%)
Female [*n* (%)]	654 (45.3%)	507 (46.2%)	147 (42.5%)
Diverse [*n* (%)]	3 (0.2%)	3 (0.3%)	0 (0%)
Length of stay on intensive care unit (days) [median (IQR)	2 (1–3)	2 (1–3)	2 (1–3)
mean (95% CI)]	3.4 (3.0–3.8)	3.5 (3.1–3.9)	3.2 (2.3–4.0)
Mechanical ventilation [*n* (%)]	259 (17.9%)	198 (18.0%)	61 (17.6%)
Duration of mechanical ventilation (days) [median (IQR)	1 (1–3)	1 (1–3)	1 (1–2)
mean (95% CI)]	3.3 (2.5–4.1)	3.7 (2.6–4.7)	2.2 (1.5–2.8)
Vasopressors [*n* (%)]	101 (7.0%)	78 (7.1%)	23 (6.7%)
Resuscitation [*n* (%)]	48 (3.3%)	38 (3.5%)	10 (2.9%)
Anticonvulsives [*n* (%)]	54 (3.7%)	44 (4.0%)	10 (2.9%)
Died [*n* (%)]	13 (0.9%)	9 (0.8%)	4 (1.2%)
Time to death (days) [median (IQR)	3 (1–3)	3 (1–3)	2.5 (1.5–9)
mean (95% CI)]	4.1 (3.0–3.8)	3.6 (1.1–6.0)	5.3 (0–15.7)
Poor outcome (GOS 1 or 2) [*n* (%)]	15 (1.0%)	11 (1.0%)	4 (1.2%)

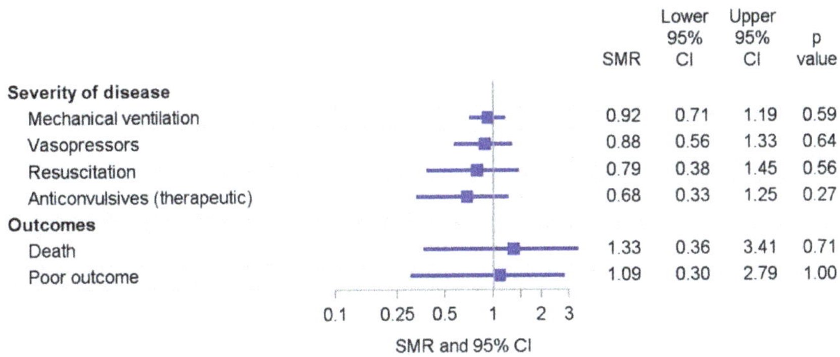

Figure 3. Trends in severity of disease and outcomes. SMR, standardized morbidity rate; CI, confidence interval.

During the lockdown period the number of PICU admissions declined from an average of 366 in 2017–2019 to 346 admissions (SMR 0.95 (95% CI 0.85–1.05)). Subgroup analyses revealed shifts in causes of admissions (Figure 3, Table 2): drowning accidents (1.36 (0.44–3.18) and ingestions (1.31 (0.81–2.01)) increased, whereas aspirations (0.71 (0.38–1.21)), burns (0.78 (0.56–1.06)), and intoxications (0.71 (0.53–0.93)) decreased. Admissions due to and trauma showed slight changes (1.07 (0.93–1.23), respectively). Within the type of trauma, we observed increases in household (1.33 (1.06–1.66)) and leisure accidents (1.34 (1.06–1.67)) that were accompanied by decreases in school/kindergarten (0.26 (0.05–0.75)) and traffic accidents (0.77 (0.57–1.02)).

The number of non-accidental injuries was lower than expected (SMR 0.68 (0.49–0.92)) (Figure 4). The overall SMR for confirmed suicide attempts was 0.68 (0.49–0.92). Stratification showed that confirmed suicide attempts increased only in adolescent males (SMR 1.38 (0.51–3.02)) and decreased in adolescent females (SMR 0.56 (0.32–0.79)) (Figure 5). Suicide attempts at ages < 12 were reported in 2 cases during the reference period and 2 cases during the lockdown and were part of extended suicide attempts.

Table 2. Types of accidents.

	Overall *n* (%)	Reference Period (2017–2019) *n* (%)	2020 *n* (%)
Type of accident			
Aspiration [*n* (%)]	68 (4.7%)	55 (5.0%)	13 (3.8%)
Burn/scalding [*n* (%)]	200 (13.9%)	159 (14.5%)	41 (11.9%)
Drowning/suffocation [*n* (%)]	16 (1.1%)	11 (1.0%)	5 (1.5%)
Ingestion [*n* (%)]	69 (4.8%)	48 (4.4%)	21 (6.1%)
Intoxication [*n* (%)]	272 (18.8%)	220 (20.0%)	52 (15%)
Inhalation of toxic gas [*n* (%)]	4 (0.3%)	3 (0.3%)	1 (0.3%)
Electrical injury [*n* (%)]	10 (0.7%)	9 (0.8%)	1 (0.3%)
Trauma [*n* (%)]	802 (55.5%)	590 (53.7%)	212 (61.3%)
Traffic [*n* (%)]	235 (29.3%)	187 (31.7%)	48 (22.6%)
Household [*n* (%)]	260 (32.4%)	180 (30.5%)	80 (37.7%)
Window fall [*n* (% of household accidents)]	64 (25.6%)	45 (25.6%)	19 (25.7%)
Leisure/sports [*n* (%)]	258 (32.1%)	178 (30.2%)	80 (37.7%)
School/kindergarten/work [*n* (%)]	38 (4.7%)	35 (5.9%)	3 (1.4%)
Unknown trauma [*n* (%)]	11 (1.4%)	10 (1.7%)	1 (0.5%)
Unknown accident [*n* (%)]	4 (0.3%)	3 (0.3%)	0 (0.0%)
Non-accidental injury [*n* (%)]			
Confirmed [*n* (%)]	223 (15.4%)	182 (16.6%)	41 (11.8%)
Confirmed and suspected [*n* (%)]	282 (19.5%)	226 (20.6%)	56 (16.2%)
Non-accidental non-suicidal	87 (6.0%)	70 (6.4%)	17 (4.9%)
Suicide attempt			
Confirmed [*n* (%)]	158 (10.9%)	129 (11.8%)	29 (8.4%)
Confirmed and suspected [*n* (%)]	184 (12.7%)	145 (13.2%)	39 (11.3%)

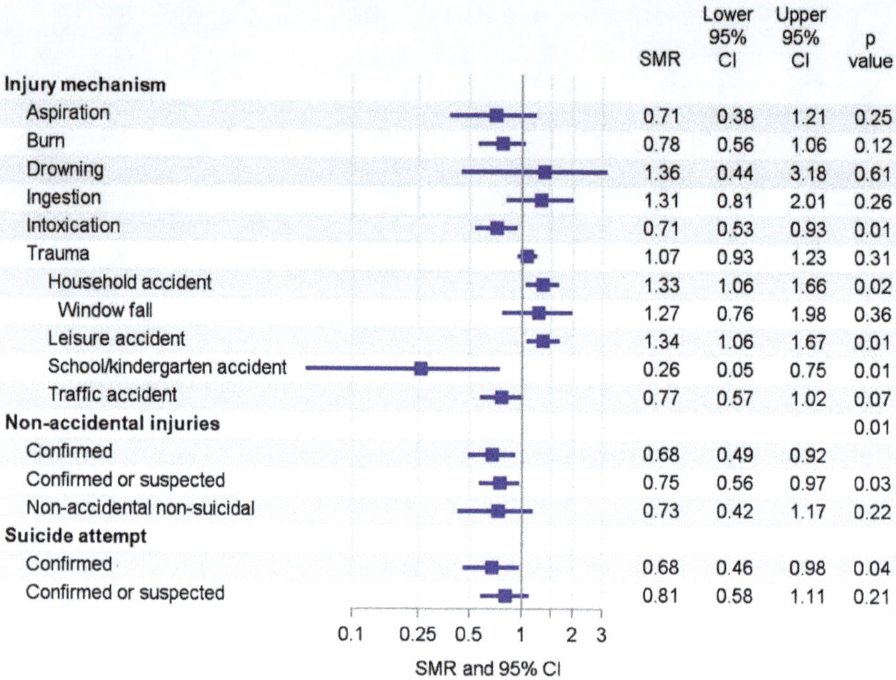

Figure 4. Trends in types of accidents. SMR = standardized morbidity rate, CI = confidence interval.

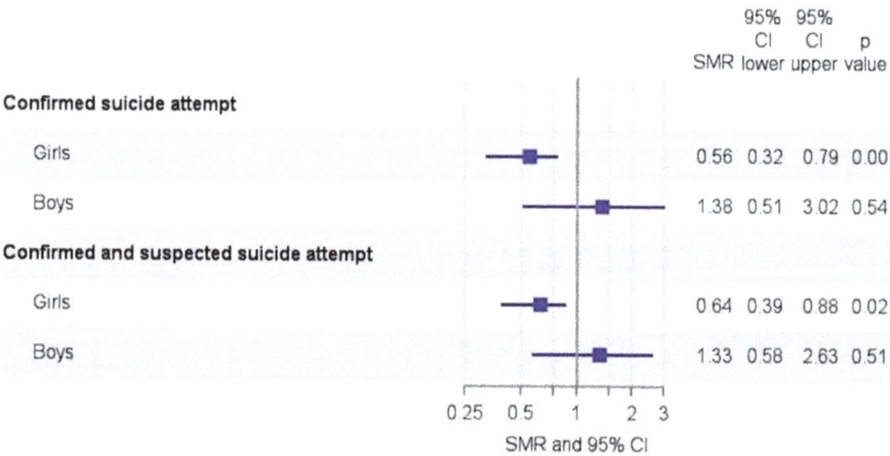

Figure 5. Trends in confirmed and suspected suicide attempts in adolescents. SMR, standardized morbidity rate; CI, confidence interval.

We observed no changes in injury patterns (Figure 6 and Table 3). The total number of patients receiving any surgery or invasive intervention averaged 124 in the reference period and was 121 during the lockdown. However, the procedures and surgeries that were performed changed: surgeries on the head (non-neurosurgery) (0.67 (0.29–1.31)) and neurosurgeries (0.69 (0.38–1.16)) declined, while at the same time surgeries to visceral organs (2.09 (1.19–3.39)) and endoscopies after ingestions or aspirations (1.18 (0.77–1.73)) increased.

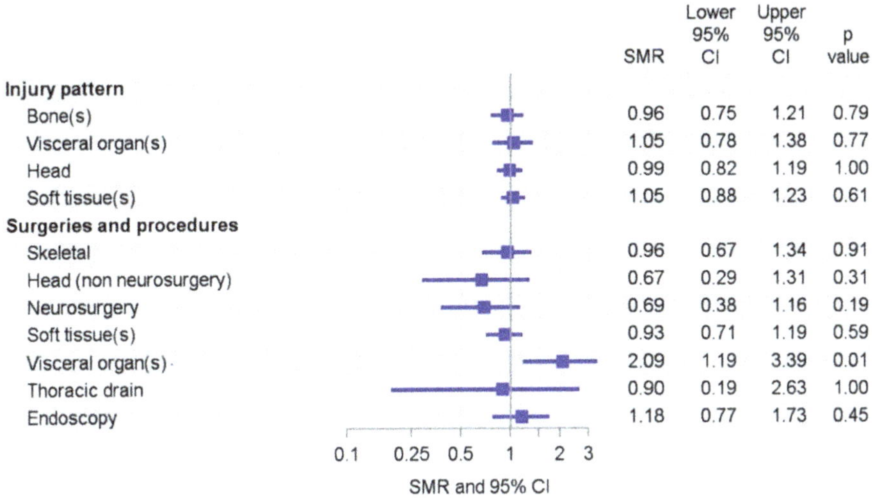

Figure 6. Trends in injury patterns and procedures. SMR = standardized morbidity rate, CI = confidence interval.

Table 3. Injury patterns and procedures.

	Overall *n* (%)	Reference Period (2017–2019) *n* (%)	2020 *n* (%)
Injury pattern			
Skeletal injury [*n* (%)]	305 (21.1%)	231 (21.0%)	74 (24.3%)
Head injury [*n* (%)]	483 (33.4%)	363 (33.0%)	120 (34.7%)
Visceral organ injury [*n* (%)]	193 (13.4%)	143 (13.0%)	50 (14.5%)
Soft tissue injury [*n* (%)]	559 (38.7%)	415 (37.8%)	144 (41.6%)
Surgeries and procedures			
Skeletal surgery [*n* (%)]	140 (9.7%)	106 (9.7%)	34 (9.8%)
Head surgery (non-neurosurgery) [*n* (%)]	44 (3.1%)	36 (3.3%)	8 (2.3%)
Neurosurgery [*n* (%)]	108 (7.5%)	88 (8.0%)	20 (5.8%)
Soft tissue procedures/surgery [*n* (%)]	265 (18.4)	203 (18.5%)	62 (17.9%)
Visceral organ surgery [*n* (%)]	39 (2.7%)	23 (2.1%)	16 (4.6%)
Thoracic drain placement [*n* (%)]			
Endoscopy (after aspiration/ingestion (*n* = 137)) [*n* (%)]	92 (67.2%)	66 (64.1%)	26 (76.5%)
Any procedure/surgery [*n* (%)]	494 (34.2%)	373 (34.0%)	121 (35.0%)

4. Discussion

In spring 2020, countries around the world faced lockdowns to control the spread of the SARS-CoV virus. Lockdown measures varied between countries, including almost complete curfews (e.g., in France and Spain). In Germany, restrictions to the normal life of children included closures of schools, daycare, sports facilities, and playgrounds and the urge to reduce social contacts. Nevertheless, children and adolescents were allowed to leave the house at any time. These drastic restrictions in the social life of children affected almost all parts of daily life, likely leading to "collateral damage" of the fight against the pandemic.

Here, we report the results of a multicenter study on PICU admissions due to accidents and injuries under the circumstances of a rather moderate lock down in Germany. We found that, in general, the number of PICU admissions due to accidents and injuries was slightly reduced compared to the same time period of the preceding years. Yet, in some aspects of trauma and injuries we could demonstrate shifts in PICU admissions during the lockdown.

As expected, we observed a reduction in school and kindergarten accidents as well as in traffic accidents. This is quite easy to explain, since only children of parents who worked in indispensable jobs, such as nurses and doctors, were allowed to attend schools and kindergartens.

Probably due to more time spent at home, household accidents increased. This increase could not be attributed to a single injury mechanism such as burns or window drops.

Several studies reported reduced pediatric health care contacts, emergency department (ED) presentations, admissions, and pediatric intensive care admissions in Italy, the UK, Scotland, and Australia during local lockdowns [2,10–13], mainly driven by substantial reductions in respiratory diseases. Trauma-specific investigations from several countries (UK, Ireland, Canada, New Zealand) showed decreases up to 60% for pediatric trauma presentations to EDs [4,14–18]. During lockdowns, children with fractures were younger and more likely to have lower limb fractures, while the total number of referrals also decreased [15]. These findings are contrary to our results. Possibly, the different lockdown types caused these discrepancies; in other countries, outdoor sports activities were restricted almost completely. One can speculate that the closure of sports facilities but unrestricted outdoor activities in Germany led to more time of unsupervised activities in children, leading to an increase in leisure accidents. It also remains speculative if the increase in leisure accidents explains the increase in abdominal surgeries. The reduction in neurosurgeries is likely caused by less severe traumatic brain injuries, as previously reported in adults [19].

Public concerns in Germany were that the reduction of social contacts would affect the psycho-emotional stability of families, leading to an increase in domestic violence and child abuse. The data from our study do not support this theory with respect to child abuse. We found a decline in non-accidental non-suicidal injuries requiring intensive care. During the lockdown, referrals reported by children's hospitals and child protection services in Germany and the UK dropped [20,21]. In France, where a strict lockdown was carried out, the number of admissions for child abuse remained unchanged among young children [22]. Self-reports by German mothers showed a considerable prevalence of 6.6% for child corporal punishment during the lockdown [23] and the prevalence of self-reported psychological and physical abuse were 8.2% and 2.4%, respectively, among Norwegian adolescents. On the other hand, a Dutch study found no differences in violence against children in families recruited before and during the lockdown. In summary, from our data and published evidence, it can neither be deduced nor reliably refuted that severe child abuse increased during the first lockdown.

Besides child abuse, children's and adolescents' mental health has received increased attention during the pandemic. PICUs are affected by changes in this field, since they are frequently involved in stabilizing patients' vital functions and surveillance after self-harm and suicide attempts. During the lockdown, psychiatric ED visits declined, as well as self-reported suicide plans or attempts [24–26]. Our study also found a decline in suicide attempts for adolescent girls, but an increase among adolescent boys. Numbers were low to draw definite conclusions, but maybe protective mechanisms such as increased feeling of belongingness and social connectedness came into effect among girls during the lockdown but not in boys.

Our study has several limitations. During the first pandemic wave, there was a gradient of higher SARS-CoV incidence rates in the south towards lower rates in the north. From the less-affected north, only few centers participated in the study, while there was clear regional clustering of participating PICUs around the main study site in Essen. Therefore, the results cannot be interpreted in a population-based manner despite the high proportion of participating PICUs. Due to the retrospective study design, PICU admission criteria were not standardized between the different centers. The study is based on the assumption that no fundamental changes in admission practice occurred in the participating PICUs between the refence period and the observation period. However, the German health care system did not collapse during the first pandemic wave and no triage was performed for acute cases and emergencies. In the pediatric sector, no restrictions or reallocation of resources was performed. PICUs were not burdened by pediatric COVID cases and did not have to care for adult COVID patients. Therefore, we assume that admission practices remained stable throughout the study period and that the results of this study are valid.

The experience from this study underlines the ability of multicenter studies to identify important epidemiologic trends over time. Prospective observational registries (e.g., the German Neonatal Network (GNN) and the British Pediatric Intensive Care Admission network (PICAnet)), have proven that they promote research that impacts clinical practice and helps to identify important trends [27–29]. German pediatric intensive care could considerably benefit from a similar PICU registry that would enable large-scale observational research in critically ill children and quality control between PICUs.

5. Conclusions

This analysis of cases from more than one fifth of the German pediatric intensive care capacities is the first study to show that, during the rather moderate German lockdown, the total burden of accident- and injury-related PICU admissions slightly declined. A decrease in school and traffic related injuries was outbalanced by an increase in household and leisure injuries. Changed trauma mechanisms entailed different surgeries compared to the pre-lockdown period. We found no evidence supporting the concern that severe child abuse increased during the lockdown. The decrease in suicide attempts among adolescent girls aligns with international reports, but the trend towards more suicide attempts in adolescent boys has not been reported. This demands verification and—if true—additional support offered to this group during future lockdowns.

Author Contributions: Study design: Study design: N.B. (Nora Bruns), C.D.-S., and U.F.-M.; data acquisition: L.Y.W., K.H. (Katharina Holtkamp), F.H., J.B., H.S., F.E., H.F. (Holger Freymann), R.H., C.A., M.H. (Michael Heldmann), J.P., D.K., A.S. (Anja Schumann), M.M.-K., N.M., C.D., P.D., T.R., M.O., K.S., F.D., F.I., F.N., P.J., M.M., N.B. (Nicole Braun), F.B.N., M.E., K.H. (Konrad Heimann), G.K.W., D.W., S.H., H.F. (Hans Fuchs), N.A., F.K., M.D. (Martin Dercks), O.K., M.D. (Marcel Dudda), J.R., and M.H. (Marc Hoppenz); statistical analyses and interpretation: N.B. (Nora Bruns), C.D.-S., A.S. (Andreas Stang), and B.K.; figures: N.B. (Nora Bruns); writing of the manuscript: N.B. (Nora Bruns), critical revision of the manuscript: all authors. All authors have read and agreed to the published version of the manuscript.

Funding: The study received funding from the Stiftung Universitätsmedizin Essen. N.B. (Nora Bruns) received funding from the Medical Faculty of the University of Duisburg-Essen (IFORES program) and from the Stiftung Universitätsmedizin Essen.

Institutional Review Board Statement: The study was conducted according to the guidelines of the Declaration of Helsinki and approved by the ethics committee of the Medical Faculty of the University of Duisburg-Essen (20-9560-BO) on 9 September 2020. Local ethics committees of the participating centers additionally approved of the study if required by local legislation.

Informed Consent Statement: Patient or legal guardian consent was not necessary according to local legislation.

Data Availability Statement: The dataset generated for this study will be made available to any qualified researcher upon reasonable request.

Conflicts of Interest: The authors declare that the research was conducted in the absence of any commercial or financial relationships that could be construed as a potential conflict of interest.

References

1. AL van Tilburg, M.; Edlynn, E.; Maddaloni, M.; van Kempen, K.; Díaz-González de Ferris, M.; Thomas, J. High Levels of Stress Due to the SARS-CoV Pandemic among Parents of Children with and without Chronic Conditions across the USA. *Children* **2020**, *7*, 193.
2. Charlesworth, J.E.G.; Bold, R.; Pal, R. Using ICD-10 diagnostic codes to identify 'missing' paediatric patients during nationwide COVID lockdown in Oxfordshire, UK. *Eur. J. Pediatr.* **2021**, *180*, 3343–3357. [PubMed]
3. Kruizinga, M.D.; Peeters, D.; van Veen, M.; van Houten, M.; Wieringa, J.; Noordzij, J.G.; Bekhof, J.; Tramper-Stranders, G.; Vet, N.J.; Driessen, G.J.A. The impact of lockdown on pediatric ED visits and hospital admissions during the COVID19 pandemic: A multicenter analysis and review of the literature. *Eur. J. Pediatr.* **2021**, *180*, 2271–2279. [PubMed]

4. Hamill, J.K.; Sawyer, M.C. Reduction of childhood trauma during the COVID-19 Level 4 lockdown in New Zealand. *ANZ J. Surg.* **2020**, *90*, 1242–1243. [CrossRef] [PubMed]
5. Van Aert, G.J.J.; van der Laan, L.; Winter, L.J.M.B.; Berende, C.A.S.; de Groot, H.G.W.; van Hensbroek, P.B.; Schormans, P.M.J.; Winkes, M.B.; Vos, D.I. Effect of the COVID Pandemic During the First Lockdown in the Netherlands on the Number of Trauma-Related Admissions, Trauma Severity and Treatment: The Results of a Retrospective Cohort Study in a Level 2 Trauma Centre. *BMJ Open* **2021**, *11*, e045015. [CrossRef]
6. McGinty, E.E.; Presskreischer, R.; Anderson, K.E.; Han, H.; Barry, C.L. Psychological Distress and COVID–Related Stressors Reported in a Longitudinal Cohort of US Adults in April and July 2020. *JAMA* **2020**, *324*, 2555. [CrossRef] [PubMed]
7. Ravens-Sieberer, U.; Kaman, A.; Erhart, M.; Devine, J.; Schlack, R.; Otto, C. Impact of the COVID pandemic on quality of life and mental health in children and adolescents in Germany. *Eur. Child Adolesc. Psychiatry* **2021**, 1–11. [CrossRef]
8. Liddell, F.D. Simple exact analysis of the standardised mortality ratio. *J. Epidemiol. Community Health* **1984**, *38*, 85–88. [CrossRef] [PubMed]
9. Uitenbroek, D.G. Sisa—Simple Interactive Statistical Analysis. Rate Ratio/SMR Exact. Available online: https://www.quantitativeskills.com/sisa/statistics/smr.htm (accessed on 3 July 2021).
10. Hu, N.; Nassar, N.; Shrapnel, J.; Perkes, I.; Hodgins, M.; O'Leary, F.; Trudgett, C.; Eapen, V.; Woolfenden, S.; Knight, K.; et al. The impact of the COVID pandemic on paediatric health service use within one year after the first pandemic outbreak in New South Wales Australia—A time series analysis. *Lancet Reg. Health West. Pac.* **2021**, *19*, 100311.
11. Raffaldi, I.; Castagno, E.; Fumi, I.; Bondone, C.; Ricceri, F.; Besenzon, L.; del Prever, A.B.; Capalbo, P.; Cosi, G.; Felici, E.; et al. Pediatric admissions to emergency departments of North-Western Italy during COVID pandemic: A retrospective observational study. *Lancet Reg. Health Eur.* **2021**, *5*, 100081. [CrossRef]
12. Rusconi, F.; Di Fabrizio, V.; Puglia, M.; Sica, M.; De Santis, R.; Masi, S.; Gagliardi, L. Delayed presentation of children to the emergency department during the first wave of COVID-19 pandemic in Italy: Area-based cohort study. *Acta Paediatr.* **2021**, *110*, 2796–2801. [CrossRef] [PubMed]
13. Williams, T.C.; MacRae, C.; Swann, O.V.; Haseeb, H.; Cunningham, S.; Davies, P.; Gibson, N.; Lamb, C.; Levin, R.; McDougall, C.M.; et al. Indirect effects of the COVID pandemic on paediatric healthcare use and severe disease: A retrospective national cohort study. *Arch. Dis. Child.* **2021**, *106*, 911–917. [PubMed]
14. Baxter, I.; Hancock, G.; Clark, M.; Hampton, M.; Fishlock, A.; Widnall, J.; Flowers, M.; Evans, O. Paediatric Orthopaedics in Lockdown: A Study on the Effect of the SARS-CoV Pandemic on Acute Paediatric Orthopaedics and Trauma. *Bone Jt. Open* **2020**, *1*, 424–430. [CrossRef] [PubMed]
15. Darling, J.; Nowicka, M.; Niazi, N.; Pillai, A. The effect of COVID lockdowns on paediatric lower limb orthopaedic presentations. *Arch. Orthop. Trauma. Surg.* **2021**, 1–8. [CrossRef] [PubMed]
16. Gilmartin, S.; Barrett, M.; Bennett, M.; Begley, C.; Ni Chroinin, C.; O'Toole, P.; Blackburn, C. The effect of national public health measures on the characteristics of trauma presentations to a busy paediatric emergency service in Ireland: A longitudinal observational study. *Ir. J. Med. Sci.* **2021**, 1–7. [CrossRef] [PubMed]
17. Keays, G.; Freeman, D.; Gagnon, I. Injuries in the time of COVID. *Health Promot. Chronic Dis. Prev. Can.* **2020**, *40*, 336–341. [CrossRef]
18. Sugand, K.; Park, C.; Morgan, C.; Dyke, R.; Aframian, A.; Hulme, A.; Evans, S.; Sarraf, K.M.; Baker, C.; Bennett-Brown, K.; et al. Impact of the COVID pandemic on paediatric orthopaedic trauma workload in central London: A multi-centre longitudinal observational study over the "golden weeks. " *Acta Orthop.* **2020**, *91*, 633–638. [CrossRef]
19. Grassner, L.; Petr, O.; Warner, F.M.; Dedeciusova, M.; Mathis, A.M.; Pinggera, D.; Gsellmann, S.; Meiners, L.C.; Freigang, S.; Mokry, M.; et al. Trends and Outcomes for Non-Elective Neurosurgical Procedures in Central Europe During the COVID Pandemic. *Sci. Rep.* **2021**, *11*, 6171.
20. Garstang, J.; Debelle, G.; Anand, I.; Armstrong, J.; Botcher, E.; Chaplin, H.; Hallett, N.; Morgans, C.; Price, M.; Tan, E.E.H.; et al. Effect of COVID lockdown on child protection medical assessments: A retrospective observational study in Birmingham, UK. *BMJ Open* **2020**, *10*, e042867. [CrossRef]
21. Heimann, T.; Ewert, J.; Metzner, F.; Sigmund, F.; Jud, A.; Pawils, S. Medical Child Protection During the Coronavirus Lockdown. *Monatsschr Kinderheilkd* **2021**, *169*, 346–352. [CrossRef]
22. Loiseau, M.; Cottenet, J.; Bechraoui-Quantin, S.; Gilard-Pioc, S.; Mikaeloff, Y.; Jollant, F.; François-Purssell, I.; Jud, A.; Quantin, C. Physical Abuse of Young Children During the COVID Pandemic: Alarming Increase in the Relative Frequency of Hospitalizations during the Lockdown Period. *Child Abuse Negl.* **2021**, *122*, 105299. [CrossRef] [PubMed]
23. Ebert, C.; Steinert, J.I. Prevalence and risk factors of violence against women and children during COVID, Germany. *Bull. World Health Organ.* **2021**, *99*, 429–438. [CrossRef] [PubMed]
24. Davico, C.; Marcotulli, D.; Lux, C.; Calderoni, D.; Cammisa, L.; Bondone, C.; Rosa-Brusin, M.; Secci, I.; Porro, M.; Campanile, R.; et al. Impact of the COVID Pandemic on Child and Adolescent Psychiatric Emergencies. *J. Clin. Psychiatry* **2021**, *82*, 31960. [CrossRef] [PubMed]
25. Koenig, J.; Kohls, E.; Moessner, M.; Lustig, S.; Bauer, S.; Becker, K.; Thomasius, R.; Eschenbeck, H.; Diestelkamp, S.; Gillé, V.; et al. The Impact of COVID Related Lockdown Measures on Self-Reported Psychopathology and Health-Related Quality of Life in German Adolescents. *Eur. Child Adolesc. Psychiatry* **2021**, 1–10. [CrossRef]

26. Ougrin, D. Debate: Emergency mental health presentations of young people during the COVID-19 lockdown. *Child Adolesc. Ment. Health* **2020**, *25*, 171–172. [CrossRef]
27. Härtel, C.; Paul, P.; Hanke, K.; Humberg, A.; Kribs, A.; Mehler, K.; Vochem, M.; Wieg, C.; Roll, C.; Herting, E.; et al. Less invasive surfactant administration and complications of preterm birth. *Sci. Rep.* **2018**, *8*, 8333. [CrossRef]
28. Humberg, A.; Dzietko, M.; Schulz, S.; Felderhoff-Müser, U.; Hüning, B.; Stein, A.; Fortmann, M.I.; Marissen, J.; Rausch, T.K.; Herting, E.; et al. Association of ApoE Genotypes and Recovery From Intracerebral Hemorrhage in Very Low Birth Weight Infants. *Stroke* **2022**, *53*, 514–522. [CrossRef]
29. Kanthimathinathan, H.K.; Buckley, H.; Davis, P.J.; Feltbower, R.G.; Lamming, C.; Norman, L.; Palmer, L.; Peters, M.J.; Plunkett, A.; Ramnarayan, P.; et al. In the eye of the storm: Impact of COVID pandemic on admission patterns to paediatric intensive care units in the UK and Eire. *Crit. Care* **2021**, *25*, 399. [CrossRef]

children

MDPI

Article

Suicidality Prevalence in a Pediatric Psychiatric Clinic: Relation to Social and Environmental Risk Factors

Stavroula Ilia [1,2,†], Evangelia Sakapeti [1,3,†], Panagiotis Briassoulis [2,4], George Gerostergios [3], Alexandros Vgontzas [3] and George Briassoulis [1,2,*]

1 Postgraduate Program "Emergency and Intensive Care in Children Adolescents and Young Adults", School of Medicine, University of Crete, 71003 Heraklion, Greece
2 Pediatric Intensive Care Unit, University Hospital, School of Medicine, University of Crete, 71110 Heraklion, Greece
3 Department of Psychiatry, University Hospital, School of Medicine, University of Crete, 71110 Heraklion, Greece
4 Attikon University Hospital, School of Medicine, National and Kapodistrian University of Athens, 12462 Athens, Greece
* Correspondence: briasoug@uoc.gr; Tel.: +30-2810-394675
† These authors contributed equally to this work.

Abstract: Suicidality is a growing public health problem in children and adolescents. The aim of this retrospective data analysis study was to estimate the prevalence of suicidality in pediatric patients admitted to an academic Pediatric Psychiatric Clinic (PPC) and to analyze social and environmental risk factors associated with suicide. Suicidal ideation was assessed by the Self-Injurious Thoughts and Behaviors Interview. Using established psychometric scales, social and stressful events were analyzed. During the four-year study, 249 episodes of care were experienced by 152 individuals (mean age 15.2 ± 2 years, girls/boys 107/45). Twenty-eight patients (11.2%) were admitted from the Pediatric Intensive Care Unit and the Department of Pediatrics, 162 (65.1%) from the Pediatric Emergency Department, and 59 (23.7%) from other Hospitals ($p = 0.003$). A significant longitudinal increase in admissions to PPC, with increasing trends of suicidal ideation, suicide attempts, and suicidality, was recorded. Suicidal behavior, bullying, internet addiction, friends quarreling, and family problems were risk factors for suicide attempts and suicidality. Our results have implications for prevention programs, highlighting an increasing need for care for suicide attempts and suicidal ideation, related to specific stressful events and contextual socio-environmental status.

Keywords: children; pediatrics; pediatric intensive care; critical care; psychiatric; suicidality; stressful; social; stress

1. Introduction

Suicidality is defined by the American Psychological Association as "the risk of suicide, usually indicated by suicidal ideation or intent, especially as evident in the presence of a well-elaborated suicidal plan, including suicidal thoughts, plans, gestures, or attempts [1]". Suicidal ideation refers to thoughts of death. The severity of suicidal ideation can vary from fleeting and unwanted thoughts to a preoccupation with death that may involve detailed planning [2].

Suicide is a leading cause of death in youth worldwide and the second cause among children and adolescents 10–24 years old. In a 5-year retrospective study of psychiatric hospitalizations of adolescents, half of the participants had experienced stressful events during childhood, with the most frequent admission reasons being aggressive behavior in males and suicide risk in females [3]. Associations between traumatic events and suicidal behavior could be used to develop more personalized intervention strategies aimed at improving mental and behavioral health of adolescents [4]. In addition, depression and anxiety in children positively predicted their suicide ideation [5].

An increase in admissions has been also recorded, affecting adolescents with suicidality/self-harm and substance-related disorders [6]. Importantly, 78.2% of adolescent admissions were due to suicidal behavior associated with family risk factors and life stressors [7]. The coronavirus disease 2019 (COVID-19) pandemic is a recent example of a mental threat to vulnerable populations, especially children and adolescents [8]. Increased psychological stress during the pandemic was associated with an increased risk of active suicidal ideation and its severity [9]. Longitudinally, the pandemic influenced the type and complexity of mental health problems, increasing the diversity and severity of suicidal behaviors and the frequency of counseling for psychotic symptoms [10]. The presence of passive suicidal ideation has been recently reported in 10.5% of 9-year-old children [11]. A recent study in children 9–10 years old demonstrated that high family conflict and low parental monitoring were associated with suicidal ideation, suicide attempts, and non-suicidal self-injury [12].

Over the past decade, visits to American and Canadian psychiatric emergency departments for child and youth life-threatening concerns have increased substantially [13]. In a 5-year period in a Pediatric Psychiatric Clinic (PPC) in Italy, a higher admission rate for females was recorded, with an average age of 13.4 years. Most of the admissions occurred through the Pediatric Emergency Department (PED), and suicidal behavior was the most frequent reason for admissions [14]. During a prolonged economic crisis, overall suicide mortality rates in Greece have increased by 40%, and Crete has been highlighted as the island with the most worrying increase, with females showing the highest rise [15,16].

Under current circumstances, investigating PPC admissions might be a noble and interesting direction for challenging research. We hypothesized that it would be of great importance to investigate the prevalence of active suicidal ideation, suicide attempts, and their associated risk factors in such a high-risk population with the aim of preventing an expanding life-threatening public health concern. Accordingly, the purpose of this study was: (1) to study suicide-related admissions in pediatric patients admitted to a PPC through the PED, Pediatric Intensive Care Unit (PICU), or other departments; (2) to analyze individual, familial, social, and environmental risk factors and their relations to suicidality in this cohort of patients; (3) to assess recent stressful events and longitudinal trends of suicide attempts, active suicidal ideation, and overall suicidality in a 4-year period.

2. Materials and Methods

2.1. Study Design

This retrospective data analysis research was conducted in the PPC, located in an academic Hospital, responsible for treating psychiatric emergencies. The sample was constituted of all children and adolescents (age 5–18-years-old) who accounted for acute hospitalizations in the PPC from February 2015 to September 2018. Exclusion criteria were patients younger than 5 or older than 18-years-old; those who did not have a parent who completed the Network of Relationships Inventory or relevant psychometric scales; and patients with parents who were not sufficiently fluent in Greek. Additionally, patients who presented with non-suicidal self-injury (NSSI) were admitted to the surgical departments and excluded from this study.

2.2. Setting

The mental health inpatient unit at the PPC in Heraklion, Crete, is an accredited facility that accommodates ten patients aged 5–18-years-old suffering from major mental, psychological, emotional disorders, and/or behavioral alterations that cannot be treated in an outpatient setting. Medical or life-threatening complications due to acute psychiatric conditions are initially managed in the PICU; patients are transferred to the PPC when stable. Upon discharge, the patient is sent back home with a consultation of the referring pediatric psychiatrist to maintain an uninterrupted treatment.

2.3. Ethical Approach

Anonymity was ensured and patients' names were replaced by a unique identification number. This study was conducted in accordance with the principles of the Declaration of Helsinki (World Medical Association Declaration of Helsinki, 1964) and was not sponsored by any pharmaceutical company. This study received ethical approval from the Institutional Review Board of the University Hospital (ID 11927/12/9/2014). Formal patient and/or parental consent was waived by the review board—in view of the retrospective and anonymized analysis of the data.

2.4. Patients

For each patient enrolled in the study, de-identified demographic, social, and psychopathological data were recorded. Age, gender, educational and school performance (cumulative grade point average), history of a previous mental health disorder, social problems, and history of physical or sexual abuse were collected. Parental disorders, including psychiatric diseases or addictions, and parents' relationship were also recorded. Data from reports of pediatric psychiatrists and psychologists were added. The following data were collected by reviewing medical records: admission reason; modality (voluntary or involuntary); outset of psychiatric pathology and recent life stressful events as previously described; the presence of suicidal ideation, suicide attempt, suicide attempt method, aggressive behavior, family, friends, and social environment. Longitudinal trends in suicidality rates were assessed by sex and age group (5–10, 11–14, and 15–18-years-old).

2.5. Suicidality

In this study, suicidality covered active suicidal ideation (serious thoughts about taking a patient's own life, suicide plans) and suicide attempts. Suicidal ideation was assessed upon admission by the Self-Injurious Thoughts and Behaviors Interview [17].

2.6. Recorded Psychometric Scales

Recorded responses to established psychometric scales about social behavior, family structure, and lifetime use of illegal drugs [18] were recorded from the medical records. Any lifetime use of illegal drugs was established for each substance separately. Then, for the needs of this study, use of tobacco was defined as smoking at least six cigarettes per day in the last 30 days; use of alcohol was defined as drinking at least 10 times in the last 30 days; use of cannabis was defined as reporting any use in the last 30 days; any lifetime use of tranquillizers and sedatives without prescription was defined as the use of available commercial names of tranquillizers and sedatives; use of any other illegal drug was defined as any lifetime use of cocaine or heroin, ecstasy, crack, amphetamines, and hallucinogens [18]. Stressful events such as migration; bullying; abuse of any etiology; and family, friend, or school problems were analytically documented. The "antisocial behavior" consisted of a 10-item scale of frequencies relating to causing damage to property, being involved in fights, and theft in the last year. The socio-economic status (total household net income, parental education and occupation, and material wealth) was collected from the patients' demographic records and recoded into three categories (high, middle, and low) [19].

A patient who had fulfilled any five of the following reported eight adapted criteria—using the internet as a means of regulating mood; putting a job or relationship in jeopardy to use the internet; lying to others about how much time is spent online; irritability, depression, or mood lability when internet use is limited; repeated efforts to curtail internet use; preoccupation with the internet; staying online longer than anticipated; and a need for increased time spent online to achieve the same amount of satisfaction—was regarded as internet-addicted [20]. Information regarding the parent–child relationship was taken from the answers to the Network of Relationships Inventory, which was used to assess quality using a 13-item short form [21]. The inventory scales of the form assess the extent to which attachment behaviors, caregiving behaviors, companionship, affiliative behaviors, conflicts, antagonism, and criticism occur in the parent–child relationships.

2.7. Associated Predictors

The associated predictors analyzed were family or school stressful events, quarreling with friends, bullying, internet addiction, physical or sexual abuse, substance abuse, and clinical or social environment and characteristics. Parental disorders, including psychiatric diseases or addictions, and parents' relationships were also recorded. Parental psychiatric diagnoses were identified based on at least two outpatient or one inpatient claims records, based on the International Classification of Diseases (tenth revision (ICD-10)) codes [22]. Parents diagnosed with any psychiatric disorder, such as schizophrenia, bipolar spectrum disorders, depressive disorders, anxiety disorders, obsessive–compulsive disorder, attention deficit hyperactivity disorder, autism spectrum disorder, adjustment disorders, and substance use disorders, were defined as having a psychiatric disorder. Parents' relationships were recorded from family social interviews, as biological parents who remained married, biological parents who divorced, step-parents, and unmarried biological parents. Data from reports of pediatric psychiatrists and psychologists were added.

2.8. Statistical Analysis

To calculate an adequate sample size, we used the G*Power statistical power calculator: chi-squared test fixed effects; power = 0.80, alpha = 0.05, effect size medium (f = 0.3). The calculated total sample size was 143. Repeated power analysis of ANOVA fixed effects, one-way; power = 0.80, alpha = 0.05, effect size medium (f = 0.3). The calculated total sample size for the cluster measurements was 195 records. The Shapiro–Wilk test was used to assess the normality of the distribution. Categorical variables are described in absolute values and frequency. Quantitative variables are expressed in mean and standard deviation. For each variable, the frequency of occurrence in the corresponding sample set was calculated. An ANOVA test was used to compare quantitative variables, and the chi-squared test, corrected by Fisher's exact test, was used for statistically significant differences in the frequencies of all variables by admission year, age group, gender, and suicidality or suicidal attempt. A logistic regression model (backward stepwise (Likelihood Ratio) method) was adopted to examine whether any of the studied risk factors are independently associated with suicidality. To evaluate risk factors' independent prediction ability, the areas under the receiver operating characteristic curves (AUROC) for risk factors significantly associated with suicide attempts were calculated. Data were analyzed by using the SPSS v.28 statistical package. Statistical significance was set at $p < 0.05$.

3. Results

3.1. Patients

A total of 249 admissions of 152 individuals (mean age 15.2 $\pm$ 2 years, mean length of stay 24 $\pm$ 31 days) were recorded and studied. One-hundred and fifty-two (61%) were first admissions and ninety-seven (39%) were repeat hospitalizations. Twenty-eight patients (11.2%) were admitted from the Pediatric Intensive Care Unit and the Department of Pediatrics, one-hundred and sixty-two (65.1%) from the Pediatric Emergency Department, and fifty-nine (23.7%) from other Hospitals ($p = 0.003$). A longitudinal increase in admissions to the PPC was recorded from 2015 to 2018 ($p < 0.03$), especially in the 15–18-year-old group (Figure 1).

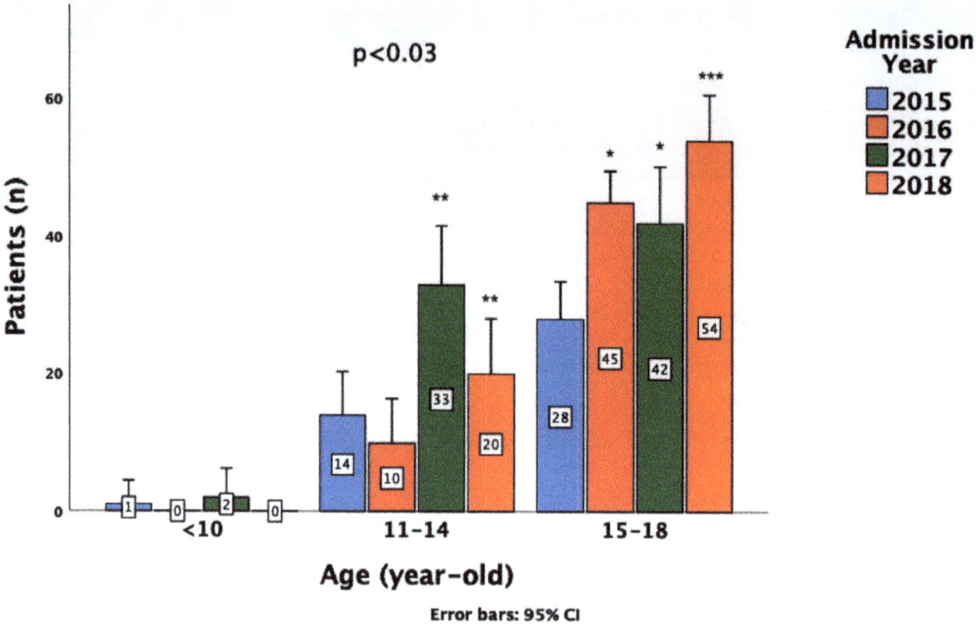

Figure 1. Longitudinal trends of admissions to the Pediatric Psychiatric Clinic per age group (ANOVA test, $p < 0.03$). Post hoc tests (Bonferroni, $p < 0.05$): Admission differences between * 2016 or 2017 vs. 2015; ** 2017 or 2018 vs. 2015 and 2016; *** 2018 vs. 2015, 2016, and 2017.

The reasons for admission to the PPC varied by sex ($p < 0.001$), with more than half of girls admitted for attempted suicide (26.5%) or suicidal behavior (32%), and most boys admitted for behavioral disorders (31%) and psychosis (22%) (Figure 2).

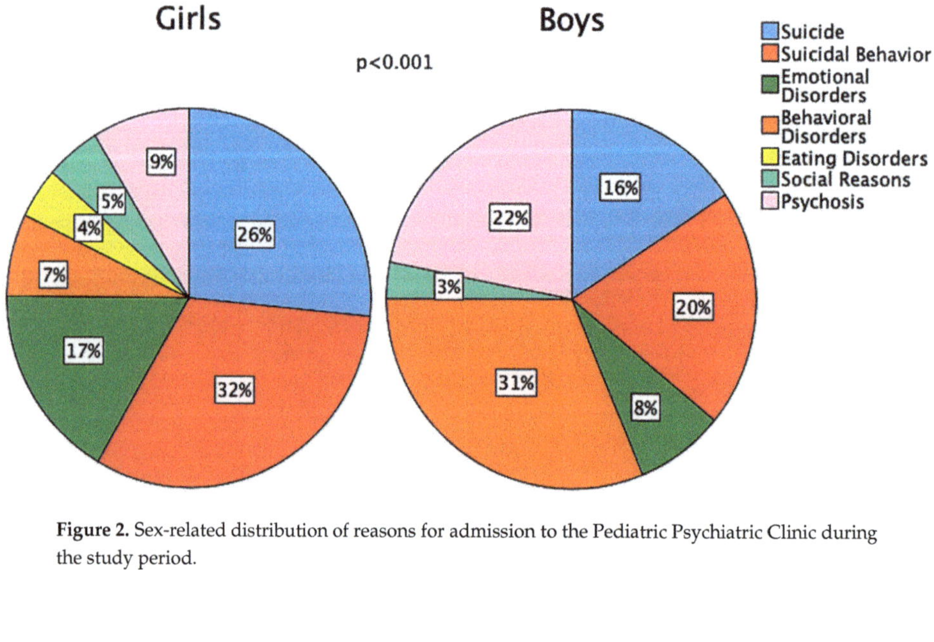

Figure 2. Sex-related distribution of reasons for admission to the Pediatric Psychiatric Clinic during the study period.

Among patients < 11-year-old, only behavioral or emotional disorders were recorded, whereas eating disorders were present only in the 11–14-year-old group ($p < 0.002$). The reasons for PPC referrals per age group, origin, admission diagnosis, and transportation conditions are shown in Table 1.

Table 1. Characteristics of acute mental health crisis episodes needing hospitalization in Pediatric Psychiatric Clinic.

Admission Characteristics			Age Group (Years)		* p
	Total	5–10	11–14	15–18	
Admission			n (%)		
First Admission	152 (61)	3 (2)	50 (32.9)	99 (65.1)	0.242
Readmission	97 (39)	0 (0.0)	27 (27.8)	70 (72.2)	
Origin					
From the Emergency Department	162 (65.1)	2 (1.2)	49 (30.3)	111 (68.5)	0.403
Another Clinic	49 (19.7)	1 (2)	17 (34.7)	31 (63.3)	
From Other Hospital	27 (10.8)	0 (0.0)	5 (18.5)	22 (81.5)	
From Outpatient Institutions	11 (4.4)	0 (0.0)	6 (54.5)	5 (45.5)	
Intra-Hospital Transport					
Pediatric Intensive Care Unit	5 (10.2)	0 (0.0)	3 (60)	2 (40)	0.003
Department of Pediatrics	23 (46.9)	1 (4.3)	14 (60.9)	8 (34.8)	
Department of Internal Medicine	12 (24.5)	0 (0.0)	0 (0.0)	12 (100)	
Department of Acute Psychiatry	9 (18.4)	0 (0.0)	0 (0.0)	9 (100)	
Admission Modality					
Voluntary	205 (82.6)	3 (1.5)	67 (32.7)	135 (65.9)	0.322
Public Prosecution Order	44 (17.3)	0 (0.0)	11 (23.3)	33 (76.7)	
Reason for Hospitalization					
Suicide Attempt	62 (24.9)	0 (0.0)	22 (35.5)	40 (64.5)	0.002
Suicidal Behavior #	72 (28.9)	0 (0)	21 (29.2)	51 (70.8)	
Emotional Disorder	33 (13.3)	1 (3.0)	8 (24.2)	24 (72.7)	
Behavioral Disorder	33 (13.3)	2 (6.1)	9 (27.3)	22 (66.7)	
Eating Disorder	8 (3.2)	0 (0.0)	8 (100)	0 (0.0)	
Social Reason	11 (4.4)	0 (0.0)	4 (36.4)	7 (63.6)	
Psychosis	30 (12.0)	0 (0.0)	5 (16.7)	25 (83.3)	

* Among age groups (ANOVA test), # evidenced at home, school, or other social environments or media.

The most common discharge ICD-10 diagnoses were emotional disorders (36.5%) and behavioral and emotional disorders with onset in childhood and adolescence (17.2%), and were associated with active suicidal ideation and suicidality ($p < 0.001$). Other less frequent diagnoses were anxiety disorder and somatoform disorders in girls, and psychotic and developmental disorders in boys ($p < 0.001$). The main reasons for readmission to PPC were attempted suicide (27%) or suicidal behavior (22.4%).

3.2. Social and Family Characteristics

The basic characteristics of patients admitted to PPC during the study period stratified by age group are presented in Table 2.

Table 2. Patients' demographics, school, family, and environmental problems, acute stressful events, and particular influencing problems.

			Age Group (Years)		* p
	Total	5–10	11–14	15–18	
(First admission data, n = 152)			n (%)		
Characteristics of patients					
Total number of patients	152 (100)	3 (2)	50 (32.9)	99 (65.1)	
Females/males	107/45 (70.4/29.6)	1/2 (0.9/4.4)	37/13 (34.6/28.9)	69/30 (64.5/66.7)	0.331

Table 2. *Cont.*

	Total	Age Group (Years)			* *p*
		5–10	11–14	15–18	
School abandonment	30 (21.5)	1 (3.3)	7 (23.3)	22 (73.3)	0.156
Family Environment					
Divorced parents	37 (30.6)	1 (2.7)	15 (40.5)	21 (56.8)	0.938
Psychiatric diseases of father or suspicion	52 (35.1)	1 (1.9)	20 (38.5)	31 (59.6)	0.423
Psychiatric diseases of mother or suspicion	98 (65.0)	1 (1)	41 (41.8)	56 (57.1)	0.018
Father's addictions	23 (15.5)	0 (0.0)	10 (43.5)	13 (56.5)	0.423
Institutions (orphanages)	22 (14.6)	0 (0.0)	6 (27.3)	16 (72.7)	0.314
(All admissions data, *n* = 249)			*n* (%)		
Recent Stressful Events					
Socio-economic status low	109 (72.7)	2 (1.8)	41 (37.6)	66 (60.6)	0.193
Problems with family relationships	77 (30.9)	1 (1.3)	24 (31.2)	52 (67.5)	0.994
Problems with school	22 (13.2)	0 (0.0)	8 (36.4)	14 (63.6)	0.819
Quarreling with friends	57 (22.9)	0 (0.0)	19 (33.3)	38 (66.7)	0.593
Bullying	60 (24.1)	0 (0.0)	26 (43.3)	34 (56.4)	0.042
Child abuse: physical	25 (10.0)	1 (4.0)	7 (28.0)	17 (68)	0.557
Child abuse: sexual	15 (6.0)	0 (0.0)	5 (33.3)	10 (66.7)	
Patient's Conditions/Addictions					
Chronic disease	68 (27.8)	1 (1.5)	20 (29.4)	47 (69.1)	0.927
Psychotic episode	50 (20.2)	0 (0.0)	12 (24)	38 (76)	0.303
Aggressive behavior	27 (10.9)	0 (0.0)	4 (14.8)	23 (85.2)	0.660
Internet addicted (patient)	91 (36.5)	2 (2.2)	28 (30.8)	61 (67.0)	0.552
Substance abuse: alcohol	6 (2.5)	0 (0.0)	1 (16.7)	5 (83.3)	0.338
Substance abuse (patient): cannabinoids	32 (13.1)	0 (0.0)	5 (15.6)	27 (84.4)	
Substance abuse (patient): other and/or more substances	6 (2.5)	0 (0.0)	1 (16.7)	5 (83.3)	

* Among age groups (ANOVA test).

More boys (36%) dropped out of abounded at school compared to girls (16%). Stressful events in the family (34.1% vs. 21.9%) mostly influenced girls ($p < 0.046$), whereas quarreling with friends did not differ between girls (24.9%) and boys (17.2%). The longitudinally-increased internet addiction (from 14.3% to 40.7%, $p = 0.016$) was most prevalent among males (32 (50%) vs. 59 (31.9%), $p < 0.08$) More girls were victims of physical (20 vs. 5) and sexual (14 vs. 1) abuse ($p = 0.03$) or bullying (26% vs. 19%) compared to boys ($p = 0.16$).

3.3. *Suicidality*

A large proportion of patients hospitalized in the PPC expressed suicidality (177/249, 71.1%). In all admissions, suicidality was more prevalent in girls (137/185, 74.1%) compared to boys (40/64, 62.5%, $p = 0.05$), with a similar trend in suicidal ideation (47% vs. 43%, $p = 0.38$) and suicide attempts (27% vs. 18.8%, $p = 0.124$). Suicidality annual rates, expressing suicide attempt rates, and active suicidal ideation longitudinal trends increased significantly ($p = 0.018$) (Figure 3).

3.4. *Risk Factors Associated with Suicidality*

Suicide attempts in the past (41.9%, $p < 0.001$) and self-harm behavior (38.3%, $p < 0.001$) were strongly associated with suicidality. Recent stressful events associated with suicidality were problems with family relationships (35.6%, $p = 0.015$), quarreling with friends (29.9%, $p < 0.001$), internet addiction (41.2%, $p = 0.02$), and bullying (32.2%, $p < 0.001$). Chronic pathologic conditions, substance abuse, physical and sexual abuse, and parental negative relations or psychiatric disorders were not related to suicidality.

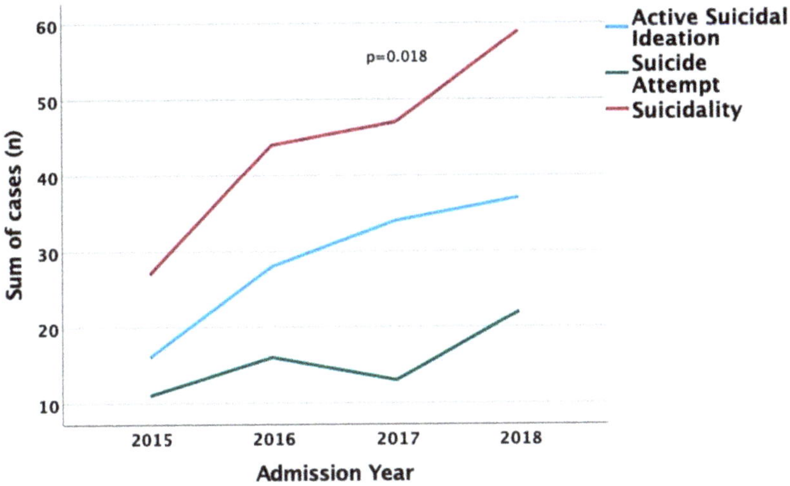

Figure 3. Suicidality, suicidal ideation, and suicide attempt annual rates during the 4-year study period.

In a logistic regression model (backward stepwise (Likelihood Ratio) method), the following risk factors were independently associated with suicidality: friends quarreling (odds ratio for suicidality 11.3, $p < 0.001$), bullying (7.4, $p = 0.001$), family problems (3.3, $p = 0.002$), and internet addiction (2.76, $p = 0.005$).

3.5. Suicide Attempt

Neither suicidality nor suicidal ideation or suicide attempts differed among age groups (Table 3). Suicide attempts recorded during the first admission ($n = 43$) or readmission ($n = 19$), along with reported previous attempts of admitted patients, gave an aggregate of 109 lifetime suicide attempts among 152 patients (71.7%) in 249 admissions (43.8%). The ways of suicide attempts did not differ between sexes, age groups, or longitudinally (Table 3).

Table 3. Suicidality, suicidal ideation, suicide attempts, and methods (all admissions).

		Age Group (Years)			* *p*
	Total	5–10	11–14	15–18	
			n (%)		
Suicidality					
Suicide attempt	62 (24.9)	0 (0.0)	22 (35.5)	40 (64.5)	0.430
Active suicidal ideation	115 (46.2)	2 (1.7)	34 (29.6)	79 (68.7)	0.721
Suicidality (both)	177 (71.1)	2 (1.1)	56 (31.6)	119 (67.2)	0.920
Suicide attempt					
First attempt at admission	43 (28.3)	0 (0.0)	16 (37.2)	27 (62.8)	0.450
Violent	23 (37.1)	0 (0.0)	12 (52.2)	11 (47.8)	0.034
Not violent	39 (62.9)	0 (0.0)	10 (25.6	29 (74.4)	
Attempt at readmission	19 (19.6)	0 (0.0)	6 (31.6)	13 (68.4)	0.560
Previous attempts ^	47 (31.3)	0 (0.0)	14 (29.8)	33 (70.2)	0.377
Suicide attempt method					
Drug overdose	35 (56.5)	0 (0.0)	9 (25.7)	26 (74.3)	0.134
Jumping from height	8 (12.9)	0 (0.0)	5 (62.5)	3 (37.5)	
Poison	4 (6.5)	0 (0.0)	1 (25)	3 (75)	
Firearm	2 (3.2)	0 (0.0)	1 (50)	1 (50)	
Wrist-cutting	3 (4.8)	0 (0.0)	3 (100)	0 (0.0)	
Drowning	2 (3.2)	0 (0.0)	0 (0.0)	2 (100)	
Vehicular impact	4 (6.5)	0 (0.0)	1 (25.0)	3 (75)	

Table 3. *Cont.*

	Age Group (Years)				* p
	Total	5–10	11–14	15–18	
Hanging	2 (3.2)	0 (0.0)	1 (50)	1 (50)	
Self-strangulation	1 (1.6)	0 (0.0)	1 (100)	0 (0.0)	
Self-immolation	1 (1.6)	0 (0.0)	0 (0.0)	1 (100)	

* Among age groups (ANOVA test), ^ before first admission.

However, younger patients more often jumped from height or cut their wrists compared to older adolescents. Patients with recorded self-harm behavior with the intention to die compared to those without the intention to die represented a significantly higher percentage in the 11–14-year-old age group (54.5%) compared to the older age group (27.5%, $p < 0.034$) and in girls (36%) compared to boys (15.3%, $p < 0.04$).

3.6. Risk Factors for Suicide Attempts

Suicide attempts in the past and self-harm behavior were not associated with a new suicide attempt. Stressful events related to suicide attempts were bullying (43.5%, $p < 0.001$), internet addiction (62.9%, $p < 0.001$), and quarreling with friends (35.5%, $p < 0.001$). The family's socioeconomic status did not correlate with the children's suicide attempts.

In an ROC analysis, suicidal behavior (sensitivity 0.97, specificity 0.61), internet addiction (sensitivity 0.63, specificity 0.73), and bullying (sensitivity 0.44, specificity 0.82) showed the strongest independent predictive ability for a suicide attempt (Figure 4).

Suicidal behavior (0.79 (95% CI = 0.73–0.84), $p < 0.001$), internet addiction (0.68 (95% CI = 0.60–0.76), $p < 0.001$), and bullying (0.63 (95% CI = 0.55–0.71), $p < 0.002$) achieved the best AUROC. Quarreling with friends was a weaker predictor of a suicide attempt (0.58 (95% CI = 0.49–0.67), $p < 0.049$).

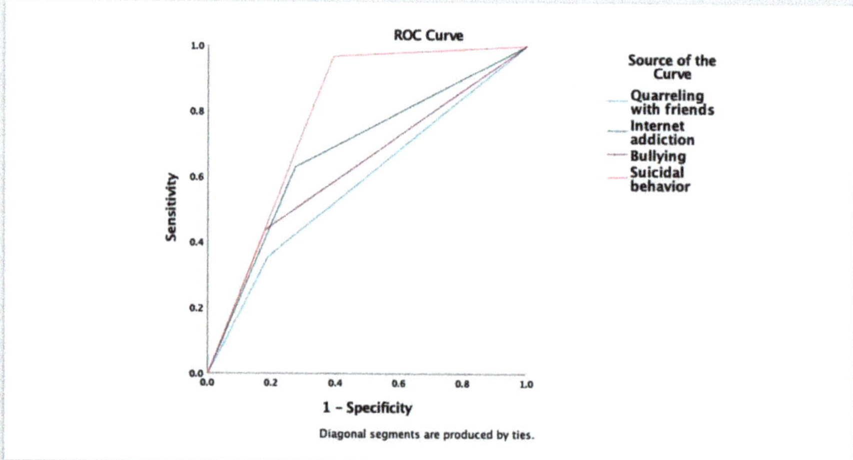

Figure 4. Area under the receiver operating characteristic curve (AUROC) for predicting suicide attempts in children and adolescents. Independently, suicidal behavior (0.79 (95% CI = 0.73–0.84), $p < 0.001$), internet addiction (0.68 (95% CI = 0.60–0.76), $p < 0.001$), and bullying (0.63 (95% CI = 0.55–0.71), $p < 0.002$) achieved the best AUROC.

4. Discussion

Our study demonstrated a longitudinal increase in annual rates of suicidality, including active suicidal ideation and suicide attempts, among patients admitted to an academic PPC. Female adolescent patients suffered mainly from suicidal ideation and were predominantly admitted for attempted suicide or active suicide ideation, whereas males were for behavioral disorders and psychosis. In our cohort of patients, we showed that suicide attempts in the past and self-harm behavior are strongly associated with suicidality, whereas the risk factors independently associated with suicidality are friend quarreling, bullying, and internet addiction. We also showed that suicidal behavior, internet addiction, and bullying are independent predictors of a suicide attempt among children and adolescents admitted to a Pediatric Intensive Care Unit or a Pediatric Emergency Department and hospitalized in an academic PPC. Unexpectedly, younger patients presented self-harm behavior with the intention to die more often compared to older adolescents.

Pediatric and adolescent patients with mental and behavioral disorders, commonly suicidality and aggressiveness, have doubled over the past 15 years. Stressors occurring over the lifespan and unhealthy family functioning play a key role in bringing psychopathology up to the surface, depicted in our study. Family functioning expresses the ability of a family to meet the physical and emotional needs of the family's members, being the most direct and predominant environment of a child's development [23]. Children and adolescents with healthy family functioning and strong family cohesion are at a low risk of developing anxiety and withdrawal behaviors. Negative family relationships, such as parent–child conflicts and divorces, increase the risk of anxiety and depressive symptoms among adolescents [24] and are associated with adolescents' internalizing problems, emotional and behavioral problems, peer problems, and conduct problems [25]. Related to the severity of family dysfunction are comorbid depression and subthreshold depressive symptoms in anxious children and adolescents [26].

The high percentages of parental psychiatric disorders in this study are supported by recent evidence, indicating that active parental psychiatric symptomatology is an established genetic–environmental factor influencing offspring psychopathology [27]. The children of parents with a mental illness may present cognitive and behavioral difficulties, resulting in poor quality of life and unhealthy social relationships [28]. Importantly, these children are at-risk of developing the same illness as their parental mental illness [29], whereas half of the children of parents with a severe mental illness are at a higher risk of developing a severe psychiatric disorder [30].

Suicide ideation prevalence, although rare in childhood, increases in adolescence and is rapidly escalated after the progression of suicide ideation to suicidal behavior. A large proportion of patients in our series expressed active suicidal ideation (46.2) or attempted suicide (24.9). Additionally, more than half of females were admitted for attempted suicide (26.5%) or active suicide ideation (32%), whereas the main reasons for readmission to PPC were attempted suicide (27%) or suicidal behavior (22.4%). Similarly, among Canadian adolescents admitted to the PICU with serious self-harm injuries, females demonstrated a higher rate of suicide attempts and prior mental health care engagement in contrast to males, who were more likely to die by suicide [31]. In similar studies, the proportion of admitted adolescents with suicide attempts was 24.5% [32], whereas admissions with suicidal behavior varied between 39% and 47%, reaching 58% in Norway [33] and 78.2% in Australia [7]. The median prevalence of any lifetime self-reported suicide attempt was 10.5% across the 17 countries that participated in the European School Survey Project on Alcohol and Other Drugs (ESPAD) 2007 school survey [19]. The finding that children < 14-years-old jump from height or cut their wrists more often than adolescents has not been reported before. Unexpectedly, in this study, children <14-years-old exhibited self-harm behavior with the intention to die more often compared to older adolescents' ways of attempting suicide. In contrast, 17.3% of admissions through the Public Prosecutor's Office in this study compare favorably to the 33% of forced admissions in the Norwegian study [33].

Suicide in adolescence has been identified as a serious public health problem worldwide. In 27 EU countries, suicide is the second cause of death among young people aged 15–19. Worryingly, the suicide rate among adolescents has increased in recent years in the USA by 24%, especially among females aged 10–14-years-old [34]. In Sweden, child suicides increased by 2.2% in each successive year from 2000 to 2018 (mean age of 16 years) [35]. Increasing trends of suicide attempts, suicidal ideation, and suicidality rates were also recorded during this 4-year study, more frequently among females and patients with self-harm behavior. These results are similar to those of a nationwide population-based study in Korea, revealing a 35.6% increase in the annual percentage change in the incidence rate of suicide-attempt-related emergency department visits over a 4-year period [36]. They have also reported that the incidence rate increase was higher among females and increased faster in mid-adolescence patients. Worryingly, during the three years of the COVID-19 pandemic (2019–2021), the number of suicide attempts by children and adolescents up to 18 years of age increased [37] along with an upward longitudinal trend of acute psychopathological symptoms, including depression, post-traumatic-stress disorder, and psychosis [10].

Stressful events related to internet addiction, bullying, and quarreling with friends were recognized as the most common predicting factors implicated in suicide attempts in this study. Similarly, in New Zealand, interpersonal conflict and relationship difficulties accounted for 50% of serious suicide attempts among young people aged 13–24, and only 6% related to school problems [38]. In our study, bullying, internet addiction, friends quarreling, and family problems were independent risk factors associated with suicidality. In a recent study among middle school students, independent risk factors associated with lifetime suicidal ideation and attempts included substance abuse and bullying victimization at school or electronically [39]. Importantly, cyberbullying experiences have recently been shown to be associated with suicidality in early adolescence [40].

Our findings that during early adolescence, suicidal children engage in problematic internet use confirm the results of a recent study showing that the problematic use of the internet and social media is independently associated with suicide attempts in young people [41]. Analyzing the changes in suicide rates after the release of "13 Reasons Why", it is now assumed that suicide increases in youth only, especially in young females, which is consistent with a contagion by media [42]. Importantly, in this and previous studies, socioeconomic status did not relate to suicide attempts, although recent studies have shown a significant impact of the financial status, fiscal austerity, and hopelessness on suicidal behavior [43,44].

The main limitations of this study are its retrospective design and the short longitudinal duration. Although the sample size is not sufficiently large to permit definitive and generalized conclusions, it is homogenous, clearly depicting various dimensions of the problem in a high-risk cohort. Future research on stressful life events and associated suicidality in children in expanded geographic areas and in the post-COVID-19 period is needed.

5. Conclusions

In the current study, we estimated the prevalence of suicidality in pediatric patients admitted to an academic Pediatric Psychiatric Clinic and analyzed social and environmental risk factors associated with suicidality. We demonstrated a longitudinal increase in active suicidal ideation and annual suicide attempt rates among patients admitted to the clinic. Female adolescent patients suffered mainly from active suicidal ideation and were predominantly admitted to the Pediatric Psychiatric Clinic, with a tenth of them to the Pediatric Intensive Care Unit, for attempted suicide or active suicidal ideation, whereas males for behavioral disorders and psychosis. We found that suicide attempts in the past and self-harm behavior were strongly associated with suicidality, whereas the risk factors independently associated with suicidality were friend quarreling, bullying, and internet addiction. We also showed that suicidal behavior, internet addiction, and bullying were independent predictors of a suicide attempt among children and adolescents. Unexpectedly, we found that younger patients presented self-harm behavior with the intention to die more often compared to older adolescents. These findings have implications for prevention and intervention programs for children and adolescents, pointing to the need for further evaluation of specific aspects of family and social life, including the COVID-19 pandemic lockdown response.

Author Contributions: Conceptualization, S.I., E.S. and G.B.; Methodology, S.I., E.S. and G.B.; Software, P.B. and G.G.; Sample collection, S.I. and E.S.; Formal analysis, S.I., P.B. and G.B.; Investigation, E.S., S.I. and G.B.; Resources: S.I., E.S., P.B., G.G., A.V. and G.B.; Writing—original draft preparation, S.I. and E.S.; Writing—review and editing, S.I., E.S., P.B., G.G. and G.B.; Supervision, A.V. and G.B.; All authors approved the final draft of the manuscript for publication. All authors have read and agreed to the published version of the manuscript.

Funding: This research received no external funding.

Institutional Review Board Statement: This study was conducted in accordance with the principles of the Declaration of Helsinki (last revised guidelines from 2013) following the International Conference on Harmonization (ICH)/Good Clinical Practice (GCP) standards for studies involving humans [28], and the Ethics Committee of the Institutional Review Board of the University Hospital approved the study (ID 11927/12/9/2014).

Informed Consent Statement: Informed consent was obtained from all subjects involved in the study.

Data Availability Statement: Clinical data presented in the study are all contained within this article. The institution's rights, including legal and ethical concerns, patient privacy, and confidentiality, restrict access to detailed data sharing.

Conflicts of Interest: The authors declare no conflict of interest.

References

1. Suicidality: Risk Factors and What You Can Do | Thriveworks. Available online: https://thriveworks.com/help-with/suicide/suicidality/ (accessed on 8 March 2023).
2. Suicidality—Anderson University. Available online: https://anderson.edu/student-life/counseling/suicidality/ (accessed on 8 March 2023).
3. Di Lorenzo, R.; Cimino, N.; Di Pietro, E.; Pollutri, G.; Neviani, V.; Ferri, P. A 5-Year Retrospective Study of Demographic, Anamnestic, and Clinical Factors Related to Psychiatric Hospitalizations of Adolescent Patients. *Neuropsychiatr. Dis. Treat.* **2016**, *12*, 191–201. [CrossRef] [PubMed]
4. Taillieu, T.L.; Sareen, J.; Afifi, T.O. Associations among Child Abuse History, Deployment-Related Traumatic Events, Mental Disorders, and Suicidal Behaviors in Canadian Regular Force Personnel. *J. Trauma. Stress* **2022**, *35*, 1060–1071. [CrossRef] [PubMed]
5. Zhang, Y.; Zhan, N.; Zou, J.; Xie, D.; Liu, M.; Geng, F. The Transmission of Psychological Distress and Lifestyles from Parents to Children during COVID-19. *J. Affect. Disord.* **2022**, *303*, 74–81. [CrossRef]
6. Bolt, J.; Patel, F.; Stone, L.; Pandian, D.; Manuel, M.M.; Gaines, N. Impact of COVID-19 on Pediatric Mental and Behavioral Health Visits to the Emergency Department. *Pediatr. Emerg. Care* **2022**, *38*, 409–415. [CrossRef] [PubMed]
7. Borschmann, R.; Stark, P.; Prakash, C.; Sawyer, S.M. Risk Profile of Young People Admitted to Hospital for Suicidal Behaviour in Melbourne, Australia. *J. Paediatr. Child Health* **2018**, *54*, 1213–1220. [CrossRef]
8. Rajkumar, R.P. COVID-19 and Mental Health: A Review of the Existing Literature. *Asian J. Psychiatr.* **2020**, *52*, 102066. [CrossRef]
9. Shi, L.; Que, J.Y.; Lu, Z.A.; Gong, Y.M.; Liu, L.; Wang, Y.H.; Ran, M.S.; Ravindran, N.; Ravindran, A.V.; Fazel, S.; et al. Prevalence and Correlates of Suicidal Ideation among the General Population in China during the COVID-19 Pandemic. *Eur. Psychiatry* **2021**, *64*, e18. [CrossRef]
10. Petruzzelli, M.G.; Furente, F.; Colacicco, G.; Annecchini, F.; Margari, A.; Gabellone, A.; Margari, L.; Matera, E. Implication of COVID-19 Pandemic on Adolescent Mental Health: An Analysis of the Psychiatric Counseling from the Emergency Room of an Italian University Hospital in the Years 2019–2021. *J. Clin. Med.* **2022**, *11*, 6177. [CrossRef]
11. Van Hove, L.; Baetens, I.; Van Leeuwen, K.; Roelants, M.; Roeljan Wiersema, J.; Lewis, S.P.; Heath, N. Passive Suicidal Ideation in Childhood. *Crisis* **2021**, *online ahead of print*. [CrossRef]
12. DeVille, D.C.; Whalen, D.; Breslin, F.J.; Morris, A.S.; Khalsa, S.S.; Paulus, M.P.; Barch, D.M. Prevalence and Family-Related Factors Associated with Suicidal Ideation, Suicide Attempts, and Self-Injury in Children Aged 9 to 10 Years. *JAMA Netw. Open* **2020**, *3*, e1920956. [CrossRef]

13. Newton, A.S.; Prisnie, K.; Macdonald, L.A.; Eltorki, M.; Finkelstein, Y.; Fitzpatrick, E.; Gagnon, I.; Greenfield, B.; Joubert, G.I.; Katz, L.Y.; et al. An Innovative Model of Pediatric Emergency Department Mental Health Care: Protocol for a Multicenter Type 1 Effectiveness-Implementation Cluster Randomized Trial. *J. Am. Acad. Child Adolesc. Psychiatry* **2022**, *61*, 946–948. [CrossRef] [PubMed]
14. Gatta, M.; Raffagnato, A.; Iannattone, S.; Mistrorigo, C.; Fasolato, R.; Traverso, A.; Zanato, S.; Miscioscia, M. Hospitalisation in Child Neuropsychiatry: A Case Study Along a Five-Year Epidemiological-Clinical Trend. *Clin. Neuropsychiatry* **2022**, *19*, 72–83. [CrossRef] [PubMed]
15. Economou, M.; Madianos, M.; Peppou, L.E.; Theleritis, C.; Patelakis, A.; Stefanis, C. Suicidal Ideation and Reported Suicide Attempts in Greece during the Economic Crisis. *World Psychiatry* **2013**, *12*, 53–59. [CrossRef] [PubMed]
16. Rachiotis, G.; Stuckler, D.; McKee, M.; Hadjichristodoulou, C. What Has Happened to Suicides during the Greek Economic Crisis? Findings from an Ecological Study of Suicides and Their Determinants (2003–2012). *BMJ Open* **2015**, *5*, e007295. [CrossRef] [PubMed]
17. Nock, M.K.; Holmberg, E.B.; Photos, V.I.; Michel, B.D. Self-Injurious Thoughts and Behaviors Interview: Development, Reliability, and Validity in an Adolescent Sample. *Psychol. Assess.* **2007**, *19*, 309–317. [CrossRef]
18. Kokkevi, A.; Richardson, C.; Olszewski, D.; Matias, J.; Monshouwer, K.; Bjarnason, T. Multiple Substance Use and Self-Reported Suicide Attempts by Adolescents in 16 European Countries. *Eur. Child Adolesc. Psychiatry* **2012**, *21*, 443–450. [CrossRef]
19. Kokkevi, A.; Rotsika, V.; Arapaki, A.; Richardson, C. Increasing Self-Reported Suicide Attempts by Adolescents in Greece between 1984 and 2007. *Soc. Psychiatry Psychiatr. Epidemiol.* **2011**, *46*, 231–237. [CrossRef]
20. Yellowlees, P.M.; Marks, S. Problematic Internet Use or Internet Addiction? *Comput. Hum. Behav.* **2007**, *23*, 1447–1453. [CrossRef]
21. Furman, W.; Buhrmester, D. The Network of Relationships Inventory: Behavioral Systems Version. *Int. J. Behav. Dev.* **2009**, *33*, 470–478. [CrossRef]
22. Jetté, N.; Quan, H.; Hemmelgarn, B.; Drosler, S.; Maass, C.; Moskal, L.; Paoin, W.; Sundararajan, V.; Gao, S.; Jakob, R.; et al. The Development, Evolution, and Modifications of ICD-10: Challenges to the International Comparability of Morbidity Data. *Med. Care* **2010**, *48*, 1105–1110. [CrossRef]
23. Dickstein, S. Family Routines and Rituals–the Importance of Family Functioning: Comment on the Special Section. *J. Fam. Psychol.* **2002**, *16*, 441–444. [CrossRef]
24. Formoso, D.; Gonzales, N.A.; Aiken, L.S. Family Conflict and Children's Internalizing and Externalizing Behavior: Protective Factors. *Am. J. Community Psychol.* **2000**, *28*, 175–199. [CrossRef] [PubMed]
25. Abu-Rayya, H.M.; Yang, B. Unhealthy Family Functioning as a Psychological Context Underlying Australian Children's Emotional and Behavioural Problems. *Internet J. Ment. Health* **2012**, *1*, 1–8.
26. Guberman, C.; Manassis, K. Symptomatology and Family Functioning in Children and Adolescents with Comorbid Anxiety and Depression. *J. Can. Acad. Child Adolesc. Psychiatry* **2011**, *20*, 186–195.
27. Biel, M.G. Parental Psychiatric Symptoms and Children's Outcomes: Toward Understanding and Responding to Intergenerational Risk in Child Psychiatry. *J. Am. Acad. Child Adolesc. Psychiatry* **2018**, *57*, 632–633. [CrossRef]
28. Reupert, A.E.; Maybery, D.J.; Kowalenko, N.M. Children Whose Parents Have a Mental Illness: Prevalence, Need and Treatment. *Med. J. Aust.* **2013**, *199*, S7–S9. [CrossRef]
29. van Santvoort, F.; Hosman, C.M.H.; Janssens, J.M.A.M.; van Doesum, K.T.M.; Reupert, A.; van Loon, L.M.A. The Impact of Various Parental Mental Disorders on Children's Diagnoses: A Systematic Review. *Clin. Child Fam. Psychol. Rev.* **2015**, *18*, 281–299. [CrossRef]
30. Rasic, D.; Hajek, T.; Alda, M.; Uher, R. Risk of Mental Illness in Offspring of Parents with Schizophrenia, Bipolar Disorder, and Major Depressive Disorder: A Meta-Analysis of Family High-Risk Studies. *Schizophr. Bull.* **2014**, *40*, 28–38. [CrossRef]
31. Mitchell, R.H.; Ani, C.; Cyr, C.; Irvine, J.; Joffe, A.R.; Skinner, R.; Wong, S.; Stang, A.S.; Laffin, M.; Korczak, D.J. Near-Fatal Self-Harm Among Canadian Adolescents. *Can. J. Psychiatry* **2021**, *67*, 598–607. [CrossRef] [PubMed]
32. Boyer, L.; Henry, J.M.; Samuelian, J.C.; Belzeaux, R.; Auquier, P.; Lancon, C.; Da Fonseca, D. Mental Disorders among Children and Adolescents Admitted to a French Psychiatric Emergency Service. *Emerg. Med. Int.* **2013**, *2013*, 651530. [CrossRef]
33. Hanssen-Bauer, K.; Heyerdahl, S.; Hatling, T.; Jensen, G.; Olstad, P.M.; Stangeland, T.; Tinderholt, T. Admissions to Acute Adolescent Psychiatric Units: A Prospective Study of Clinical Severity and Outcome. *Int. J. Ment. Health Syst.* **2011**, *5*, 1. [CrossRef]
34. Curtin, S.C.; Warner, M.; Hedegaard, H. Increase in Suicide in the United States, 1999–2014. *NCHS Data Brief.* **2016**, *241*, 1–8.
35. Junuzovic, M.; Lind, K.M.T.; Jakobsson, U. Child Suicides in Sweden, 2000–2018. *Eur. J. Pediatr.* **2022**, *181*, 599–607. [CrossRef] [PubMed]
36. Lee, K.-S.; Lim, D.; Paik, J.-W.; Choi, Y.Y.; Jeon, J.; Sung, H.K. Suicide Attempt-Related Emergency Department Visits among Adolescents: A Nationwide Population-Based Study in Korea, 2016–2019. *BMC Psychiatry* **2022**, *22*, 418. [CrossRef] [PubMed]
37. Ciccotti, H.R.; Spiller, H.A.; Casavant, M.J.; Kistamgari, S.; Funk, A.R.; Smith, G.A. Pediatric Suspected Suicides and Nonfatal Suicide Attempts Reported to United States Poison Control Centers Before and During the COVID-19 Pandemic. *J. Med. Toxicol.* **2023**, *epub ahead of print*. [CrossRef]
38. Beautrais, A.L.; Joyce, P.R.; Mulder, R.T. Precipitating Factors and Life Events in Serious Suicide Attempts among Youths Aged 13 through 24 Years. *J. Am. Acad. Child Adolesc. Psychiatry* **1997**, *36*, 1543–1551. [CrossRef] [PubMed]

39. Flores, J.P.; Stuart, E.A.; Swartz, K.L.; Jallah, N.A.; Wilcox, H.C. Risk and Protective Factors Associated with Suicidal Thoughts and Behaviors Among Maryland Middle School Students. *School Ment. Health* **2022**, *14*, 1024–1043. [CrossRef]
40. Arnon, S.; Klomek, A.B.; Visoki, E.; Moore, T.M.; Argabright, S.T.; DiDomenico, G.E.; Benton, T.D.; Barzilay, R. Association of Cyberbullying Experiences and Perpetration with Suicidality in Early Adolescence. *JAMA Netw. Open* **2022**, *5*, e2218746. [CrossRef]
41. Sedgwick, R.; Epstein, S.; Dutta, R.; Ougrin, D. Social Media, Internet Use and Suicide Attempts in Adolescents. *Curr. Opin. Psychiatry* **2019**, *32*, 534–541. [CrossRef]
42. Niederkrotenthaler, T.; Stack, S.; Till, B.; Sinyor, M.; Pirkis, J.; Garcia, D.; Rockett, I.R.H.; Tran, U.S. Association of Increased Youth Suicides in the United States with the Release of 13 Reasons Why. *JAMA Psychiatry* **2019**, *76*, 933–940. [CrossRef]
43. Bachmann, S. Epidemiology of Suicide and the Psychiatric Perspective. *Int. J. Environ. Res. Public Health* **2018**, *15*, 1425. [CrossRef] [PubMed]
44. Fang, M. School Poverty and the Risk of Attempted Suicide among Adolescents. *Soc. Psychiatry Psychiatr. Epidemiol.* **2018**, *53*, 955–967. [CrossRef] [PubMed]

children

MDPI

Article

Impact of Time Point of Extracorporeal Membrane Oxygenation on Mortality and Morbidity in Congenital Diaphragmatic Hernia: A Single-Center Case Series

Christian Wegele [1,2], Yannick Schreiner [1], Alba Perez Ortiz [1], Svetlana Hetjens [3], Christiane Otto [4], Michael Boettcher [5], Thomas Schaible [1] and Neysan Rafat [1,*]

1 Department of Neonatology, University Children's Hospital Mannheim, University of Heidelberg, 68167 Mannheim, Germany; christianwegele@web.de (C.W.); yschreiner@gmx.de (Y.S.); alba.perez-ortiz@umm.de (A.P.O.); thomas.schaible@umm.de (T.S.)

2 Department of Neonatology, Pediatric Intensive Care and Sleep Medicine, Vestische Kinder-Jugendklinik Datteln, University Witten/Herdecke, 45711 Datteln, Germany

3 Department of Biomathematics and Medical Statistics, Medical Faculty Mannheim, University of Heidelberg, 68167 Mannheim, Germany; svetlana.hetjens@medma.uni-heidelberg.de

4 Department of Obstetrics and Gynecology, University Medical Center Mannheim, University of Heidelberg, 68167 Mannheim, Germany; christiane.otto@umm.de

5 Department of Pediatric Surgery, University Children's Hospital Mannheim, University of Heidelberg, 68167 Mannheim, Germany; michael.boettcher@umm.de

* Correspondence: neysan.rafat@umm.de; Tel.: +49-(0)621-383-3510

Abstract: Since there are no data available on the influence of the time point of ECMO initiation on morbidity and mortality in patients with congenital diaphragmatic hernia (CDH), we investigated whether early initiation of ECMO after birth is associated with a beneficial outcome in severe forms of CDH. All neonates with CDH admitted to our institution between 2010 until 2020 and undergoing ECMO treatment were included in this study and divided into four different groups: (1) ECMO initiation < 12 h after birth (n = 143), (2) ECMO initiation between 12–24 h after birth (n = 31), (3) ECMO initiation between 24–120 h after birth (n = 48) and (4) ECMO initiation > 120 h after birth (n = 14). The mortality rate in the first (34%) and fourth group (43%) was high and in the second group (23%) and third group (12%) rather low. The morbidity, characterized by chronic lung disease (CLD), did not differ significantly in the three groups; only patients in which ECMO was initiated >120 h after birth had an increased rate of severe CLD. Our data, although not randomized and limited due to small study groups, suggest that very early need for ECMO and ECMO initiation > 120 h after birth is associated with increased mortality.

Keywords: congenital diaphragmatic hernia; extracorporeal membrane oxygenation; chronic lung disease

1. Introduction

Congenital diaphragmatic hernia (CDH) is characterized by the failure of diaphragmatic development and prenatal thoracic herniation of abdominal organs, leading to lung hypoplasia and persistent pulmonary hypertension of the newborn (PPHN) [1]. If conventional treatment with gentle ventilation and optimized vasoactive medication fails, extracorporeal membrane oxygenation (ECMO) may be considered [1]. Currently, CDH is the most common indication for ECMO in neonates [2], but survival rates reported by the extracorporeal life support organization (ELSO) have continued to drop in the modern era [3]. Indications for initiating ECMO include either respiratory or circulatory parameters, which are also undergoing continuous refinement. The benefits of ECMO in CDH are still controversial, and systematic reviews concerning a benefit of ECMO in CDH did not find an advantage for this therapeutic option [4–6]. However, some centers and networks have demonstrated an increase in survival rates in CDH with the employment of ECMO by retrospective analysis in their series [7,8]. However, data on long-term results, including morbidity and quality of life, are rare. Survival might be influenced by the timing of ECMO initiation and the timing of surgical repair. In this regard, a trend toward early initiation of ECMO and early surgery on ECMO exists [2]. The use of ECMO in CDH will continue to be evaluated, and prospective randomized trials and registry network are necessary to help in answering the addressed questions of patient selection and management.

We hypothesized that an early initiation of ECMO after birth is associated with a beneficial outcome in severe forms of CDH. In this study, we evaluated the impact of the timing of ECMO initiation on the clinical outcome of CDH patients.

2. Materials and Methods

2.1. *Subjects and Clinical Data*

All newborn infants with CDH treated between 1 January 2010 and 31 March 2020, who received ECMO support at our neonatal intensive care unit (NICU) at the Department of Neonatology of the University Children's Hospital Mannheim, University of Heidelberg, were included in this retrospective study. ECMO support was initiated according to the recommendations suggested by the CDH EURO Consortium Consensus and ELSO [2,9]. Exclusion criteria were patients with associated anomalies (including cardiac malformation), syndromes or chromosomal aberrations. The study population was divided into the four following groups depending on the time point of ECMO initiation: (1) ECMO initiation < 12 h after birth, (2) ECMO initiation between 12–24 h after birth, (3) ECMO initiation between 24–120 h after birth and (4) ECMO initiation 120 h after birth. The surgical correction was performed after stabilization of the neonate after ECMO in all cases. Pre-, peri- and postnatal clinical parameters were collected from the patient's records, and mortality and morbidity were compared between the groups. Morbidity was represented by duration of mechanical ventilation, duration of hospitalization and development of chronic lung disease (CLD). The diagnosis of CLD was made as reported before [10,11]: if there was an additional need for oxygenation at day 28 after birth, CLD was diagnosed. Severity of CLD was differentiated into three grades according to the additional need for oxygenation at day 56 after birth: mild CLD with no need for supplemental inspired oxygen (fraction of inspired oxygen (Fio2) ≤ 0.21), moderate CLD (Fio2, 0.22–0.29), and severe CLD (Fio2 ≥ 0.30). For some patients being discharged to other hospitals before the 56th day of life, CLD could be diagnosed, but severity could not be assessed. If outcome information was missing, patients were categorized as 'CLD n/a'. The defect size of each CDH patient was assessed according to the consensus of the CDH study group [12]. This study was approved by the local ethics committee of the Medical Faculty Mannheim of the University of Heidelberg (reference number: 2019-884R).

2.2. *Statistical Analysis*

Statistical calculations were performed using SAS software, release 9.4 (SAS Institute Inc., Cary, NC, USA). For qualitative variables, absolute and relative frequencies are given. For quantitative and approximately normally distributed variables, mean values and standard deviations were calculated. For skewed or ordinal data, minimum and maximum are presented. To compare groups regarding qualitative parameters, a Chi-square test or Fisher's exact test was used where appropriate. For normally distributed data, a one-way analysis of variance (ANOVA) was performed to compare the mean values of different age groups. For these analyses, the SAS procedure PROC MIXED was used. Adjustment for multiple comparisons was done by Scheffé test. A *p*-value of <0.05 was considered statistically significant.

3. Results

In this study, 243 patients were included. One patient was excluded because of missing data about the start of the ECMO and six patients were excluded for additional cardiac malformation. For an overview of the recruitment of CDH patients into this study and the characteristics of the dropouts, please see Supplementary Figure S1.

Of 236 analyzed patients, 145 (61.4%) were male and 91 (38.6%) were female. Further, 188 (79.7) patients presented with left-sided and 48 (20.3%) patients with right-sided CDH. Moreover, 209 (88.6%) children were diagnosed with CDH prenatally, whereas 27 (12.4%) were still unknown on delivery. For an overview of the characteristics of the study population, please refer to Table 1.

Table 1. Clinical data for each study group.

	Study Group									
	1 (n = 143)		2 (n = 31)		3 (n = 48)		4 (n = 14)		All (n = 236)	
GA (weeks)	37.3	±1.40	38.1	±1.50	38.0	± 1.68	38.0	± 0.68	37.6	±1.47
GW (g)	2915	±422	3140	±535	3035	±624	3015	±552	2975	±494
ApH	7.31	±0.1	7.30	±0.1	7.30	±0.08	7.25	±0.11	7.30	±0.07
5 min APGAR	7.31	±1.20	7.30	±1.90	7.30	±1.77	7.25	±1.16	7.07	±1.46
paO_2 6 h prior to ECMO (mmHg)	72.9	±73.0	65.3	±34.0	79.4	±53.2	77.8	±51.0	74.3	±56.1
Age at ECMO initiation (h)	5.68	±2.00	17.5	±3.60	48.1	±25.5	240	±123	29.7	±63.3
Duration of ECMO (h)	247	±105	247	±99.1	207	±76.9	208	±78.1	237	±98.6
$AaDO_2$ prior to ECMO	596	±33.1	613	±17.4	621	±18.4	604	±22.2	604	±29.9
OI prior to ECMO	36.1	±20.4	43.6	±28.6	35.6	±17.7	27.9	±14.8	36.5	±21.0
Duration of MV (d)	35.2	±33.2	36.2	±20.5	37.6	±22.9	41.4	±21.0	36.2	±29.2
Duration of hospitatlization (d)	73.5	±62.5	84.6	±70.5	90.1	±63.3	67.2	±44.8	77.7	±62.6
TFLV (%)	27.4	±10.8	28.2	±11.6	34.4	±12.8	30.6	±7.52	28.8	±11.2
o/e LHR (%)	35.0	±11.4	41.7	±20.6	37.0	±10.2	37.8	±14.1	36.2	±12.5

Data are presented in means ± standard deviation (SD). GA = gestational age, GW = gestational weight, ApH = arterial umbilical cord pH, ECMO = extracorporeal membrane oxygenation, OI = oxygenation index, TFLV = total fetal lung volume, o/e LHR = observed/expected lung-to-head-ratio.

Overall survival was 71.6%, but when looking at each group individually, survival rates differed from 66.4% (n = 95) in the first group to 77% (n = 24) in the second group, 87.5% (n = 42) in the third group and 57% (n = 8) in the fourth group, respectively (Table 2). Survival in group 2 and group 3 was significantly higher than in group 1 and group 4 (p = 0.011).

Table 2. Survival and frequencies of CDH patch, abdominal patch and liver-up phenomenon.

	Study Group				p-Value
	1 (n = 143)	2 (n = 31)	3 (n = 48)	4 (n = 14)	
Survival	0.66	0.77	0.88	0.57	**0.0110**
CDH patch	0.99	1.00	0.96	1.00	0.34
Abdominal patch	0.45	0.32	0.30	0.36	0.31
Liver-up	0.93	0.93	0.74	0.69	**0.0009**

Data are presented in percentage of each group's study population. CDH = congenital diaphragmatic hernia. The bold points out that these p-values are statistically significant.

Some clinical data were collected and compared for all the groups (Table 2). Values for $AaDO_2$ prior to ECMO initiation for group 1 versus group 2 (p = 0.035) and group 1 versus group 3 ($p < 0.0001$) were significant (Table 2). Further, liver herniation was significantly less in patients in group 3 and group 4 ($p < 0.001$) (Table 2). For the remaining clinical parameters, differences between the groups were not significant (Table 2).

When looking at parameters for ventilation and oxygenation prior to ECMO initiation, the highest pCO_2 was determined in group 1, requiring ECMO support earliest compared to the other groups. Levels of pCO_2 immediately before ECMO initiation in group 1 were significantly higher compared to group 3 ($p < 0.0001$) and marginally higher compared to group 4, respectively ($p = 0.052$) (Figure 1A). There were no significant differences between the groups concerning the level of paO_2 prior to ECMO initiation (Figure 1B).

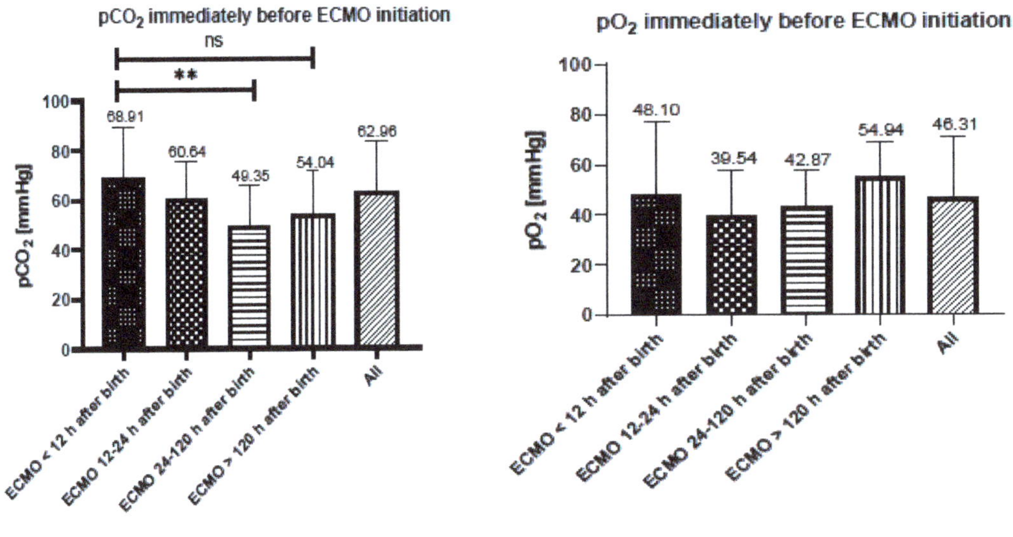

(**A**) (**B**)

Figure 1. Ventilation (**A**) and oxygenation (**B**) parameters prior to ECMO initiation. ** statistically significant. "ns" stands for not significant.

Evaluation of morbidity was performed by assessing chronic lung disease (CLD) and for this purpose, patients from group 1 and group 2 were pooled together due to the need of ECMO for the same pathophysiological reason, namely pulmonary ventilation disorder. In group 1 and 2, the incidence of CLD was significantly lower compared to the other two groups (Figure 2). CDH patients in group 3 had the highest number of mild CLD cases, whereas patients in group 4 had significantly higher numbers of moderate and severe CLD (Figure 2).

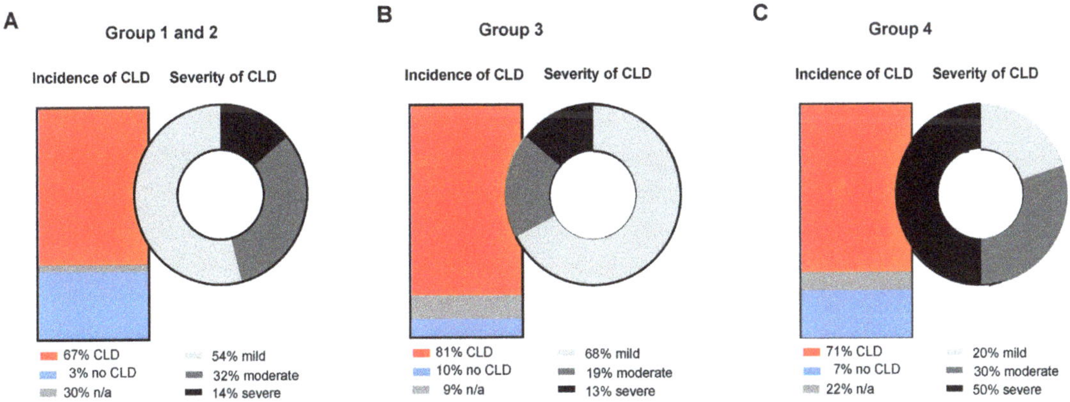

Figure 2. Incidence and severity of chronic lung disease (CLD) in the different groups of the study population: (**A**) group 1 (ECMO initiation <12 h after birth) and 2 (ECMO initiation 12–24 h after birth), (**B**) group 3 (ECMO initi ation 24–120 h after birth) and (**C**) group 4 (ECMO initiation 120 h after birth).

The defect size of each CDH patient was assessed according to the consensus of the CDH study group. There was no significant difference regarding defect size between the four different groups (Table 3).

Table 3. Frequencies of CDH defect size (A–D) according to CDH study group consensus.

		A	B	C	D	p-Value
Group	1 (n = 143)	0.01	0.09	0.65	0.25	0.46
	2 (n = 31)	0.00	0.16	0.73	0.11	
	3 (n = 48)	0.00	0.26	0.55	0.19	
	4 (n = 14)	0.00	0.14	0.72	0.14	

4. Discussion

In this study, we collected clinical parameters over a ten-year period from CDH patients undergoing ECMO, which were referred to our center. There is evidence suggesting a critical time point for ECMO initiation in patients with CDH to improve outcome. To our knowledge, this is the first report to show that CDH newborns with a later ECMO initiation, between 12 h and 120 h after birth, have a significant survival benefit compared to newborns undergoing a very early or very delayed ECMO intervention within the first 12 h or beyond 120 h of life, respectively.

4.1. Indication for ECMO in CDH

ECMO in neonates should be initiated when indication occurs. Indication in classical neonatal ECMO (e.g., meconium aspiration syndrome) is usually present when oxygenation index is above 40 [2,13]. However, in CDH, indication for ECMO is more complex [1,9]. While applying gentle ventilation for small lungs, the mean airway pressure does not exceed values over 15. Therefore, with an FiO_2 of 1.0 and arterial paO_2 below 50mmHg, where hypoxia starts to occur, OI is only 30 and may be a cut off to start ECMO in CDH [1,9].

However, in most cases, hypercarbia, not hypoxia, and metabolic acidosis trigger severe pulmonary hypertension (PHT) and an entry criterion in CDH may be a persisting pH-value below 7.15 (corresponding with $paCO_2$ values between 60 and 100 mmHg) [1,9]. In such a situation of acidosis, PHT can also be recognized as a pre-postductal saturation difference of more than ten percent.

A third indication for starting ECMO is circulatory failure, with low cardiac output, low urinary output and rising lactate [1,2,9]. However, this criterion is rare and often occurs later than hypercapnia and hypoxia. A honeymoon period occurs in those patients, in which a respiratory acidosis can be overwhelmed and pCO_2-value below 60 mmHg can be reached.

4.2. Parameters for Predicting ECMO

There are many data about prenatal parameters and prognosis [14]. To date, LHR, TFLV and liver herniation into the thoracic cavity are the most reliable prenatal predictors for mortality in CDH [15]. Likewise, liver herniation and lung volume could also predict the need for ECMO support in these patients [10]. However, the prognostic value of prenatal data is not clear and treating patients with the same disease severity may lead to different results and, therefore, it is difficult to compare treatment centers. Treatment strategies may vary even between high-volume centers and results are not the same [7].

Significantly fewer data are available for prognostic value of early postnatal parameters predicting mortality [16,17]. Of course, high OI calculated by respiratory parameters after delivery leads more often to ECMO than lower OI, and survival of CDH patients with ECMO is lower than survival of CDH patients without ECMO [18]. For example, Wilford Hall Santa Rosa Formula (highest paO_2—highest $paCO_2$ during initial 24 h of life) includes values of pCO_2 [16,19]. If the difference of the best paO_2 minus highest $paCO_2$ is below zero, there is high risk for mortality. Postnatal prognostic values of this formula are fairly high and calculation is possible as early as one hour after delivery and standardized primary care. Applying the Wilford Hall Santa Rosa Formula to our results, the value is lowest in group 1 with the poorest prognosis.

4.3. Honeymoon in CDH Prior to ECMO

A honeymoon period with higher values of oxygenation (temporarily arterial paO_2 over 60 mmHg) and vanishing pre-postductal saturation difference occurs in those patients in whom a respiratory acidosis can be overwhelmed and pCO_2-value below 60 mmHg can be reached. A honeymoon period may indicate a better responsiveness of pulmonary vessels and, therefore, a better prognosis. This scenario mostly occurs in patients from group 2 and 3 and leads to ECMO success rates of about 80%. The lower paO_2 directly before initiation of ECMO reflects the sudden end of the honeymoon period with a rebound phenomenon caused by vasoconstriction of pulmonary vessels.

Patients without a honeymoon period do not respond to treatment strategies prior to ECMO and are treated with ECMO earlier and this course leads to a poorer prognosis, with survival rates from ECMO of 66% in group 1. Looking at the basic data of these patients, they started even prenatally with the lowest values of fetal lung volume. Surprisingly, the outcome of initial honeymooners, but late decision for ECMO because of a longer apparently stable phase of several days, was poorest. This result leads one to speculate that responsiveness of pulmonary vascular bed to the unloading effect of ECMO and, therefore, the potential to overwhelm PHT in CDH decreases towards the end of the first week of life. It can be assumed that the effectiveness of the PHT treatment has become blunted.

Reaching a honeymoon by high-frequency oscillation ventilation (HFOV) may occur in some patients but one side effect of HFOV is a tendency to overdistension of the lungs and the effort of controlling $paCO_2$ often leads to hypoxemia. The VICI trial showed that HFOV ventilation seems inferior to CMV [20]. HFOV is able to control $paCO_2$ but may delay ECMO initiation and, therefore, poorer survival rates were seen in CDH patients treated with HFOV as the initial mode of ventilation [20].

4.4. Chronic Lung Disease after ECMO

The development of CLD represents an important risk factor for impaired pulmonary outcome in CDH patients. Although neonatal ECMO has improved the survival of CDH patients, improved survival might carry a higher risk of long-term morbidity among survivors [21]. There is conflicting evidence about the development of CLD in ECMO survivors. In an older prospective study, ECMO support resulted in a 50% reduction in CLD in survivors of severe respiratory failure [22]. Other studies have demonstrated that ECMO support does not prevent sequelae of severe respiratory disease in the newborn period [23]. Since lung development is already disturbed in CDH due to lung hypoplasia and pulmonary hypertension, additional risk factors, such as CLD, impair pulmonary outcome significantly.

Our study adds data concerning the pulmonary outcome defined by the severity of CLD. The risk for developing CLD is very high in group 3 and 4, and extremely high for developing severe CLD in group 4 (50%). Although patients in group 4 had a seemingly better prenatal expected prognosis in comparison to group 3 due to, e.g., less liver-up, mortality and morbidity (severe CLD) were much higher in this group. Since early ECMO initiation was associated with less mortality and severe CLD, it appears that ECMO should be started earlier, independently from the indication's parameter.

Whether persisting pulmonary hypertension or more severe lung damage with longer time on high ventilator settings are more contributable to CLD was not investigated.

5. Conclusions

Our data, although not randomized and limited due to small study groups, suggest that very early need for ECMO and ECMO initiation >120 h after birth is associated with increased mortality and even with morbidity in late ECMO initiation. Therefore, future studies have to be conducted to identify and stratify the best timepoint for initiating ECMO in the different forms of CDH, depending on prenatal risk factors for ECMO employment (e.g., fetal lung volume, liver-up, etc.) and postnatal factors (e.g., degree of PHT, acidosis, etc.).

Supplementary Materials: The following supporting information can be downloaded at: https://www.mdpi.com/article/10.3390/children9070986/s1, Figure S1: Recruitment of study population.

Author Contributions: Conceptualization, T.S. and N.R.; methodology, C.W., T.S. and N.R.; validation, A.P.O., S.H. and C.O.; formal analysis, C.W., Y.S., A.P.O., S.H. and N.R.; investigation, C.W. and Y.S.; data curation, C.W., Y.S. and N.R.; writing—original draft preparation, C.W., Y.S. and N.R.; writing—review and editing, M.B., T.S. and N.R.; visualization, Y.S.; supervision, T.S. and N.R. All authors have read and agreed to the published version of the manuscript.

Funding: This research received no external funding.

Institutional Review Board Statement: The study was conducted in accordance with the Declaration of Helsinki and approved by the local ethics committee of the Medical Faculty Mannheim of the University of Heidelberg (reference number: 2019-884R, date of approval: 19 December 2019).

Informed Consent Statement: Patient consent was not required for this type of retrospective study.

Data Availability Statement: The data presented in this study are available on request from the corresponding author.

Conflicts of Interest: The authors declare no conflict of interest.

References

1. Rafat, N.; Schaible, T. Extracorporeal membrane oxygenation in congenital diaphragmatic hernia. *Front. Pediatr.* **2019**, *7*, 336. [CrossRef]
2. Brogan, T.V.; Lequier, L.; Lorusso, R.; MacLaren, G.; Peek, G. *Extracorporal Life Support: The ELSO Red Book*, 5th ed.; Brogan, T.V., Lequier, L., Lorusso, R., MacLaren, G., Peek, G., Eds.; Extracorporeal Life Support Organization: Ann Arbor, MI, USA, 2017; ISBN 978-0-9656756-5-9.
3. Turek, J.W.; Nellis, J.R.; Sherwood, B.G.; Kotagal, M.; Mesher, A.L.; Thiagarajan, R.R.; Patel, S.S.; Avansino, J.R.; Rycus, P.T.; McMullan, D.M.; et al. Shifting risks and conflicting outcomes—ECMO for neonates with congenital diaphragmatic hernia in the modern era. *J. Pediatr.* **2017**, *190*, 163–168.e4. [CrossRef]
4. Wilson, J.M.; Lund, D.P.; Lillehei, C.W.; O'Rourke, P.P.; Vacanti, J.P. Delayed repair and preoperative ECMO does not improve survival in high-risk congenital diaphragmatic hernia. *J. Pediatr. Surg.* **1992**, *27*, 368–375. [CrossRef]
5. Wilson, J.M.; Lund, D.P.; Lillehei, C.W.; Vacanti, J.P. Congenital diaphragmatic hernia—A tale of two cities: The Boston experience. *J. Pediatr. Surg.* **1997**, *32*, 401–405. [CrossRef]
6. Azarow, K.; Messineo, A.; Pearl, R.; Filler, R.; Barker, G.; Bohn, D. Congenital diaphragmatic hernia—A tale of two cities: The Toronto experience. *J. Pediatr. Surg.* **1997**, *32*, 395–400. [CrossRef]
7. Snoek, K.G.; Greenough, A.; van Rosmalen, J.; Capolupo, I.; Schaible, T.; Ali, K.; Wijnen, R.M.; Tibboel, D. Congenital diaphragmatic hernia: 10-year evaluation of survival, extracorporeal membrane oxygenation, and foetoscopic endotracheal occlusion in four high-volume centres. *Neonatology* **2018**, *113*, 63–68. [CrossRef]
8. Schaible, T.; Hermle, D.; Loersch, F.; Demirakca, S.; Reinshagen, K.; Varnholt, V. A 20-year experience on neonatal extracorporeal membrane oxygenation in a referral center. *Intensive Care Med.* **2010**, *36*, 1229–1234. [CrossRef]
9. Snoek, K.G.; Reiss, I.K.M.; Greenough, A.; Capolupo, I.; Urlesberger, B.; Wessel, L.; Storme, L.; Deprest, J.; Schaible, T.; Van Heijst, A.; et al. Standardized postnatal management of infants with congenital diaphragmatic hernia in Europe: The CDH EURO Consortium Consensus—2015 Update. *Neonatology* **2016**, *110*, 66–74. [CrossRef]
10. Kastenholz, K.E.; Weis, M.; Hagelstein, C.; Weiss, C.; Kehl, S.; Schaible, T.; Neff, K.W. Correlation of observed-to-expected MRI fetal lung volume and ultrasound lung-to-head ratio at different gestational times in fetuses with congenital diaphragmatic hernia. *Am. J. Roentgenol.* **2016**, *206*, 856–866. [CrossRef]
11. Jobe, A.H.; Bancalari, E. Bronchopulmonary dysplasia. *Am. J. Respir. Crit. Care Med.* **2001**, *163*, 1723–1729. [CrossRef]
12. Lally, K.P.; Lasky, R.E.; Lally, P.A.; Bagolan, P.; Davis, C.F.; Frenckner, B.P.; Hirschl, R.M.; Langham, M.R.; Buchmiller, T.L.; Usui, N.; et al. Standardized reporting for congenital diaphragmatic hernia—An international consensus. *J. Pediatr. Surg.* **2013**, *48*, 2408–2415. [CrossRef]
13. Sebald, M.; Friedlich, P.; Burns, C.; Stein, J.; Noori, S.; Ramanathan, R.; Seri, I. Risk of Need for Extracorporeal membrane oxygenation support in neonates with congenital diaphragmatic hernia treated with inhaled nitric oxide. *J. Perinatol.* **2004**, *24*, 143–146. [CrossRef]

14. Oluyomi Obi, T.; Kuret, V.; Puligandla, P.; Lodha, A.; Lee-Robertson, H.; Lee, K.; Somerset, D.; Johnson, J.; Ryan, G. Antenatal predictors of outcome in prenatally diagnosed congenital diaphragmatic hernia (CDH). *J. Pediatr. Surg.* **2017**, *52*, 881–888. [CrossRef]
15. Hedrick, H.L.; Danzer, E.; Merchant, A.M.; Bebbington, M.W.; Zhao, H.; Flake, A.W.; Johnson, M.P.; Liechty, K.W.; Howell, L.J.; Wilson, R.D.; et al. Liver position and lung-to-head ratio for prediction of extracorporeal membrane oxygenation and survival in isolated left congenital diaphragmatic hernia. *Am. J. Obstet. Gynecol.* **2007**, *197*, 422.e1–422.e4. [CrossRef]
16. Hoffman, S.B.; Massaro, A.N.; Gingalewski, C.; Short, B.L. Survival in congenital diaphragmatic hernia: Use of predictive equations in the ECMO population. *Neonatology* **2011**, *99*, 258–265. [CrossRef]
17. Weis, M.; Burhany, S.; Perez Ortiz, A.; Nowak, O.; Hetjens, S.; Zahn, K.; Schoenberg, S.; Schaible, T.; Rafat, N. The chest radiographic thoracic area can serve as a prediction marker for morbidity and mortality in infants with congenital diaphragmatic hernia. *Front. Pediatr.* **2021**, *9*, 740941. [CrossRef]
18. Ruttenstock, E.; Wright, N.; Barrena, S.; Krickhahn, A.; Castellani, C.; Desai, A.P.; Rintala, R.; Tovar, J.; Till, H.; Zani, A.; et al. Best oxygenation index on day 1: A reliable marker for outcome and survival in infants with congenital diaphragmatic hernia. *Eur. J. Pediatr. Surg.* **2015**, *25*, 3–8. [CrossRef]
19. Schultz, C.M.; DiGeronimo, R.J.; Yoder, B.A. Congenital diaphragmatic hernia study group congenital diaphragmatic hernia: A simplified postnatal predictor of outcome. *J. Pediatr. Surg.* **2007**, *42*, 510–516. [CrossRef]
20. Snoek, K.G.; Capolupo, I.; van Rosmalen, J.; Hout, L.d.J.d.; Vijfhuize, S.; Greenough, A.; Wijnen, R.M.; Tibboel, D.; Reiss, I.K.M. CDH EURO consortium conventional mechanical ventilation versus high-frequency oscillatory ventilation for congenital diaphragmatic hernia. *Ann. Surg.* **2016**, *263*, 867–874. [CrossRef]
21. Perez Ortiz, A.; Glauner, A.; Dittgen, F.; Doniga, T.; Hetjens, S.; Schaible, T.; Rafat, N. Chronic lung disease following neonatal extracorporal membrane oxygenation. A single center experience. *Front. Pediatr.* **2022**. Available online: https://www.frontiersin.org/articles/10.3389/fped.2022.909862/abstract (accessed on 17 May 2022).
22. Vaucher, Y.E.; Dudell, G.G.; Bejar, R.; Gist, K. Predictors of early childhood outcome in candidates for extracorporeal membrane oxygenation. *J. Pediatr.* **1996**, *128*, 109–117. [CrossRef]
23. Beardsmore, C.; Dundas, I.; Poole, K.; Enock, K.; Stocks, J. Respiratory function in survivors of the United Kingdom extracorporeal membrane oxygenation trial. *Am. J. Respir. Crit. Care Med.* **2000**, *161*, 1129–1135. [CrossRef] [PubMed]

children

MDPI

Article

Safety and Tolerability of Continuous Inhaled Iloprost Therapy for Severe Pulmonary Hypertension in Neonates and Infants

Amit V. Krishnan [1,†], Victoria Freniere [2,†], Rakesh Sahni [3], Diana P. Vargas Chaves [3], Sankaran S. Krishnan [4], Dimitrios Savva [2,‡] and Usha S. Krishnan [1,*,‡]

1 Department of Pediatrics (Cardiology), Columbia University Irving Medical Center, New York, NY 10932, USA; akrishna@student.touro.edu
2 Department of Pharmacy, New York-Presbyterian Hospital, New York, NY 10065, USA; victoria.freniere@bmc.org (V.F.); dis9082@nyp.org (D.S.)
3 Department of Pediatrics (Neonatology), Columbia University Irving Medical Center, New York, NY 10032, USA; rs62@cumc.columbia.edu (R.S.); dv2373@cumc.columbia.edu (D.P.V.C.)
4 Department of Pediatrics, New York Medical College, Valhalla, NY 10595, USA; sankaran_krishnan@nymc.edu
* Correspondence: usk1@cumc.columbia.edu
† These authors contributed equally to this work.
‡ These authors also contributed equally to this work.

Abstract: This is a single-center retrospective study to assess the safety and tolerability of continuous inhaled iloprost use as rescue therapy for refractory pulmonary hypertension (PH) in critically ill neonates and infants. A retrospective chart review was performed on 58 infants and data were collected at baseline, 1, 6, 12, 24, 48 and 72 h of iloprost initiation. Primary outcomes were change in heart rate (HR), fraction of inspired oxygen (FiO_2), mean airway pressures (MAP), blood pressure (BP) and oxygenation index (OI). Secondary outcomes were need for extracorporeal membrane oxygenation (ECMO) and death. 51 patients treated for >6 h were analyzed in 2 age groups, neonate ($\leq$28 days: n = 32) and infant (29–365 days: n = 19). FiO_2 ($p < 0.001$) and OI ($p = 0.01$) decreased, while there were no significant changes in MAP, BP and HR. Of the fifteen patients placed on ECMO, seven were bridged off ECMO on iloprost and eight died. Twenty-four out of fifty-one patients (47%) recovered without requiring ECMO, while twelve (23%) died. Iloprost as add-on therapy for refractory PH in critically ill infants in the NICU has an acceptable tolerability and safety profile. Large prospective multicenter studies using iloprost in the neonatal ICU are necessary to validate these results.

Keywords: continuous iloprost; pulmonary hypertension; neonate; infant; outcome

1. Introduction

Pulmonary hypertension (PH) is a severe and often fatal disease, especially when it occurs in the neonatal and infant age group. PH can present as persistent pulmonary hypertension of the newborn (PPHN) in preterm or term neonates. PPHN can occur either as primary or idiopathic PPHN in about 10% neonates and secondary, in association with acute respiratory inflammation in the setting of meconium aspiration syndrome, pneumonias, hyaline membrane disease, transient tachypnea of newborn, developmental lung diseases, genetic disorders, as well as in congenital heart diseases (CHDs) [1–3]. Neonates with primary PPHN have an abnormal transition from fetal to postnatal circulation, resulting in sustained elevations of pulmonary vascular resistance and persistent hypoxemia after birth compromising hemodynamics [2,3]. Preterm infants with ongoing bronchopulmonary dysplasia (BPD) or term infants with CHD or other developmental lung disorders can present with significant and persistent PH even after the first few months of life and can have significant morbidity and mortality from PH crises in association with infection and inflammation [3,4].

Therapies for PH target the components of vascular remodeling and belong to three classes: phosphodiesterase inhibitors, endothelin receptor antagonists, and prostanoids [4–6]. Prostanoids are analogs of prostacyclin, which when bound to receptors, cause increases in cyclic adenosine monophosphate that result in a cascade of phosphorylation events that subsequently result in smooth muscle relaxation and reduced cell proliferation, thereby reducing pulmonary vascular resistance and inhibiting the remodeling associated with PH [6–13]. Although inhaled nitric oxide (iNO) is recommended as first line therapy to decrease PVR in infants with PPHN, and is the only approved PH therapy for PPHN, it does not improve survival and about 40% of neonates may fail to respond to iNO alone [7]. Epoprostenol, the first approved prostanoid medication, significantly improved long-term survival in PH patients. It has also been used successfully in neonatal PH [8,9]. Epoprostenol is administered as a continuous intravenous infusion through an indwelling central line, which is associated with a host of additional risks, such as need for access, bacteremia, sepsis, thromboembolism and rebound PH if the infusion is interrupted due to its extremely short half-life [6]. Iloprost is a more chemically stable prostaglandin analog and may be administered intermittently or continuously via inhalation. The inhaled administration specifically targets the lung vessels with less systemic effects and possibly less ventilation perfusion mismatch than intravenous epoprostenol, especially in infants with developmental lung disorders [6–13]. Iloprost peaks at 20–30 min and leaves the system within an hour after administration. Thus, continuous iloprost inhalation to prevent fluctuations in PA pressures is an attractive option.

Several adult studies and a few small pediatric studies have demonstrated favorable outcomes when patients were placed on adjunctive inhaled iloprost therapy after they had inadequate responses to current PAH therapies. Although these studies suggested some benefits, they were smaller in size, did not have a uniform population base and did not look at the effects of continuous inhaled iloprost therapy in neonates and infants [12–14]. Neonates with PH may be refractory to iNO and may rapidly deteriorate, leading to extracorporeal membrane oxygenation (ECMO) cannulation and/or death. Intravenous or inhaled prostanoids have been used to try and maintain hemodynamics by lowering the PVR in these patients and act as additional therapy to iNO [5–13,15,16]. Evidence demonstrates that inhaled iloprost therapy significantly reduces pulmonary arterial pressure and PVR with equal potency to iNO with minimal systemic side effects within the pediatric population with CHD [11,14]. Little is known about the safety and efficacy of inhaled iloprost in the neonatal and infant population. The use of continuous iloprost in older children has recently been described [10]. The aim of this study is to evaluate the safety, tolerability and outcomes, including ECMO and death after continuous inhaled iloprost in infants with refractory PH in the NICU. We also describe the institutional practices for medication dosing, delivery, titration and wean of inhaled continuous iloprost therapy.

2. Materials and Methods

This is a single-center retrospective observational study of neonates and infants admitted to the NICU at Morgan Stanley Children's Hospital of New York Presbyterian. Patients were included if they received iloprost therapy between February 2020 and May 2023. Patients < 1 year of age with the 6th World Symposium of Pulmonary Hypertension (6th WSPH) Groups I and III PH were included, while patients with Group II PH (left heart disease and pulmonary vein stenosis) and Group V PH with complex congenital heart disease were excluded. This study was approved by the Columbia University Irving Medical Center's Institutional Review Board and electronic medical and pharmacy records were queried to identify patients and collect data. Since our new electronic Medical Record system, Epic, was implemented in February 2020, we could only consistently obtain data from this date and beyond.

Demographic data included age and weight at iloprost start, gestational age, birth weight, Apgar scores, iloprost dose and duration, iNO dose, inotropes, other PH medications, steroid administration, level of ventilatory support, need for ECMO, underlying diagnosis associated with PH, and outcomes. Additionally, fraction of inspired oxygen (FiO_2), mean airway pressure (MAP), partial pressure of arterial oxygen (PaO_2), mean blood pressure (mBP), heart rate (HR) and oxygen index ((OI) = $FiO_2 \times MAP/PaO_2$) were collected at baseline, 1, 6, 12, 24, 48 and 72 h after initiation of iloprost therapy. The vasoactive inotrope score (VIS) was calculated using the doses of inotropes at the time of iloprost start (Dopamine dose + Dobutamine dose + 100 × Epinephrine dose + 10 × Milrinone dose + 100 × Norepinephrine dose (all in mcg/kg/minute) + 10,000 × Vasopressin dose (U/kg/min)) [17,18].

2.1. *Method of Administration*

Inhaled iloprost was only used in infants with severe persistent PH despite treatment with iNO and other PH therapy. A test dose of iloprost (2.5 mcg) was administered over 20 min to assess for hypotension or worsening in oxygenation. If the initial iloprost dose was well tolerated, continuous therapy was initiated. Iloprost was administered through the inhalation tubing port closest to the endotracheal tube (to reduce dead space) and occasionally extra diluent was provided to prevent crystallization or clogging of the tube. The treatment dose range of iloprost was between 1 and 7.5 mcg/h. Our weaning protocol consisted of a gradual reduction in the dosage to 1 mcg/h. This was followed by weaning to intermittent iloprost with bolus dosing at gradually prolonged intervals up to every four hours until discontinuation. Primary outcomes included change in FiO_2, MAP, OI, HR and mBP from baseline to 72 h. Secondary outcomes included the need for ECMO or death during iloprost therapy. The reason for stopping iloprost and side effects were documented.

The data were analyzed as a whole, and patients were separated into two groups—neonates (<28 days) and infants (28–365 days)—as the etiology of PH and the frailty of the patients are different in the two groups.

2.2. *Statistical Analysis*

The data were analyzed using SPSS version 16 for Windows. Binomial and categorical data were analyzed by chi-squared and Fisher's exact test. Non-parametrically distributed continuous data were analyzed by the Mann–Whitney U test. Continuous variables were not assumed to be normally distributed, so values were reported as medians with interquartile range (IQR) provided. A p value of <0.05 was considered significant. Friedman's two-way ANOVA by ranks was used to evaluate distributions of measured pulmonary and systemic respiratory and hemodynamic markers (FiO_2, MAP, OI, mean BP, HR) over time, with a p value of <0.05 considered significant.

3. Results

3.1. *Demographics*

A cohort of fifty-one patients with the sixth WSPH Group I or III PH who were treated with inhaled iloprost as rescue therapy were analyzed. Seven additional patients received iloprost for <6 h and were not included in the analysis. The patients ranged from 0 to 310 days old, and their weights ranged from 2.9 to 4.3 kg. Within this cohort, 31 patients survived, while 20 died. Fifteen patients required ECMO during their hospital course. Thirty-two patients ≤28 days of age at the time of treatment were categorized into the neonate group and the remaining nineteen patients ≥28–365 days of age at time of treatment were categorized into the infant group. Thirty-one neonates were ≤10 days of age, while one patient was 21 days old with a diagnosis of surfactant protein deficiency. In the neonate group, PH was secondary to congenital heart disease (CHD) in 10 patients, and congenital diaphragmatic hernia (CDH) in nine. Other causes of PH in this group included meconium aspiration, hypoxic ischemic encephalopathy, sepsis and developmental lung diseases. The infants were 41–310 days old at time of iloprost therapy and had a diagnosis of CHD in 12, CDH in three, and BPD in four. Gender differences in demographics and clinical characteristics of the study population are described in Table 1. There were no statistically significant differences in demographics, clinical characteristics, and outcomes between male and female neonates.

Table 1. Demographic and clinical characteristics of the study population stratified by sex.

	Number of Patients (%)	Male (%)	Female (%)	p *
Total	51 (100%)	30	21	
Neonate	32 (62.7%)	17 (56.7%)	15 (71.4%)	0.28
Need for ECMO	15 (29.4%)	8 (26.7%)	7 (33.3%)	0.61
Mortality	20 (39.2%)	14 (46.7%)	6 (28.6%)	0.19
	Total (range)	Male (IQR)	Female (IQR)	p **
Median Birth Weight (kg)	3.080 (0.375–4.420)	3.13 (2.320–3.380)	3.08 (2.550–3.300)	0.69
Median Gest. Age (Weeks)	38.57 (23–41)	37.57 (35.71–39.00)	38.71 (37.14–39.14)	0.28
Median Weight at Iloprost Admin. (kg)	3.37 (2.06–7.3)	3.43 (2.99–4.38)	3.30 (2.97–3.71)	0.70
Apgar Score 1¢	6.00 (2.00–8.00)	5.00 (2.50–7.00)	7.00 (3.00–8.00)	0.25
Apgar Score 5¢	8.00 (7.00–9.00)	7.00 (7.00–8.50)	8.00 (7.00–9.00)	0.50
VIS	13.00 (0–19.00)	13.00 (3.50–16.80)	13.00 (6.00–20.00)	0.62
Iloprost # Days	3.00 (0.25–37)	3.00 (1.00–8.80)	3.00 (1.00–7.00)	0.76

* chi-squared test; ** Mann–Whitney test.

There was a significantly greater proportion of neonates in our sample compared to infants (Table 2). There was also a difference in gestational age (the BPD patients in the infant group had a lower gestational age and presented with severe PH later), weight at time of iloprost dosing, and in VIS between the two groups. Two infants with critical PH had a VIS of 0. This was secondary to vasoactive medications being discontinued after being cannulated on ECMO.

Table 2. Outcomes in neonates and infants with PH treated with iloprost (n = 51).

	Neonate (%)	Infant (%)	p *
Total	32 (62.7%)	19 (37.3%)	**0.01**
Male	17 (53.1%)	13 (68.4%)	0.28
ECMO	12 (37.5%)	3 (15.8%)	0.12 **
Deceased	13 (40.6%)	7 (36.8%)	0.79
	median (IQR)	Median (IQR)	p ***
Birth Wt (kg) (range)	3.195 (0.540–4.29)	3.05 (0.375–4.42)	0.52
Gest. age (weeks)	39.00 (37.14–39.14)	37.00 (30.14–38.79)	**0.02**
Weight at iloprost administration (kg)	3.21 (2.75–3.38)	4.53 (3.77–5.56)	**<0.01**
Apgar score 1¢	5.00 (2.75–8.00)	6.50 (2.75–8.00)	0.74
Apgar score 5¢	7.00 (6.50–9.00)	8.00 (7.00–9.00)	0.55
VIS	14.50 (6.75–23.13)	5.00 (0.00–14.50) *	**0.03**
Iloprost # days	1.00 (1.00–5.50)	3.00 (1.00–10.00)	0.07

* chi-squared test; ** Fischer's exact test; *** Mann–Whitney test. Bold indicates significance.

3.2. Other PH Medications

All patients were on 20 PPM iNO, 12 patients received sildenafil, four received sildenafil and bosentan (dual therapy), nine in the neonate group were on prostaglandin E1 (to keep the ductus arteriosus patent) and three were on parenteral epoprostenol, which was weaned off when iloprost was initiated. Inotropes at the time of iloprost start included milrinone (32), epinephrine (30), vasopressin (19), dopamine (9), dobutamine (6) and norepinephrine (5), demonstrating the severity of hemodynamic compromise among these children.

There was a significantly greater proportion of patients in our sample who were not cannulated to ECMO compared to patients who did (Table 3). There was a significant difference in Apgar scores at 5 min between ECMO and non-ECMO patients, but none of the other parameters achieved significance.

Table 3. Characteristics of patients requiring vs. not requiring ECMO cannulation.

	ECMO (%)	**No ECMO (%)**	p *
Total	15 (29.4%)	36 (70.6%)	**<0.01**
Male	8 (53.3%)	22 (61.1%)	0.61
Neonate	12 (80.0%)	20 (55.6%)	0.12 **
Deceased	7 (46.7%)	13 (36.1%)	0.48
	ECMO (IQR)	No ECMO (IQR)	p ***
Birth Wt (kg)	3.08 (2.49–3.28)	3.13 (2.50–3.39)	0.88
Gest. Age (weeks)	38.57 (37.14–39.00)	38.21 (35.67–39.00)	0.88
Dosing Wt (kg)	3.22 (2.72–3.71)	3.51 (3.20–4.13)	0.10
Apgar score 1¢	6.00 (4.50–8.00)	5.00 (2.00–8.00)	0.23
Apgar score 5¢	9.00 (7.00–9.00)	7.00 (5.00–8.00)	**0.04**
VIS	15.00 (4.50–22.50)	10.50 (3.75–15.63)	0.22
Iloprost # days	2.00 (1.00–14.50)	3.00 (1.00–7.25)	0.55

* chi-squared test; ** Fisher's exact test; *** Mann–Whitney test. Bold indicates significance.

There was a significant difference in the proportion of patients who survived compared to the proportion of patients who died while on iloprost in our sample (Table 4). No other differences were observed between surviving and deceased patients.

Table 4. Characteristics of patients who survived vs. deceased patients.

	Survived (%)	**Deceased (%)**	p *
Total	31 (60.8%)	20 (39.2%)	**0.03**
Male	16 (51.6%)	14 (70.0%)	0.19
Neonate [<4 wk age]	19 (61.3%)	13 (65.0%)	0.79
ECMO	8 (25.8%)	7 (35.0%)	0.48
	Survived (IQR)	Deceased (IQR)	p **
Birth Wt (kg)	3.20 (2.50–3.58)	3.06 (2.41–3.28)	0.32
Gest. age (weeks)	39.00 (37.00–39.14)	37.29 (35.71–38.89)	0.23
Dose Wt (kg)	3.70 (3.21–4.41)	3.22 (2.75–3.61)	0.06
Apgar score 1¢	6.00 (3.00–8.00)	5.00 (2.50–7.50)	0.83
Apgar score 5¢	8.00 (7.00–9.00)	7.00 (7.00–9.00)	0.59
VIS	11.00 (3.00–16.50)	14.00 (6.00–21.25)	0.40
Iloprost # days	3.00 (1.00–10.00)	1.50 (0.94–6.75)	0.48

* chi-squared test; ** Mann–Whitney test. Bold indicates significance.

3.3. Improvement in Parameters over the Evaluated Time Period

Friedman's two-way analysis of variance was performed to detect significant changes in FiO_2, OI, MAP, mean BP and HR over the 72 h study period. FiO_2 ($p < 0.001$) and OI

($p = 0.01$) decreased over the study period, suggesting improved oxygenation (Figure 1a,c). Supplementary Figure S1a,c show similar improvements in the patients who did not need ECMO.

(a)

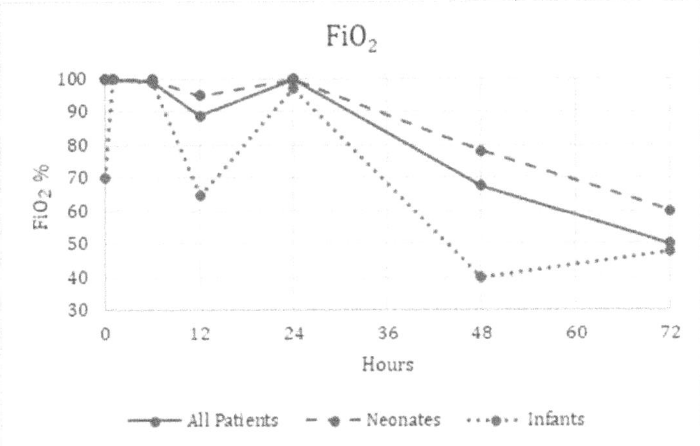

(b)

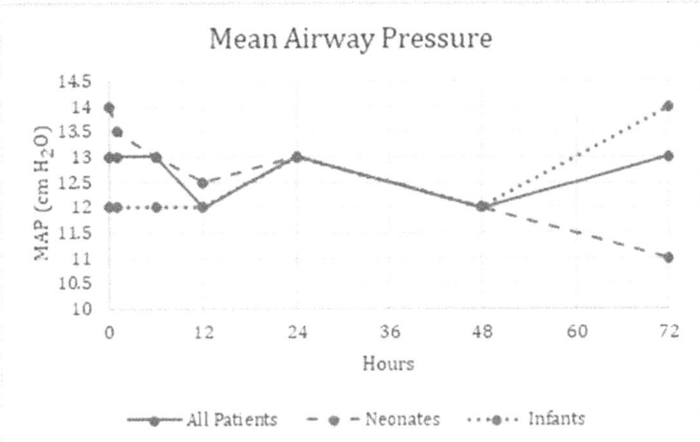

(c)

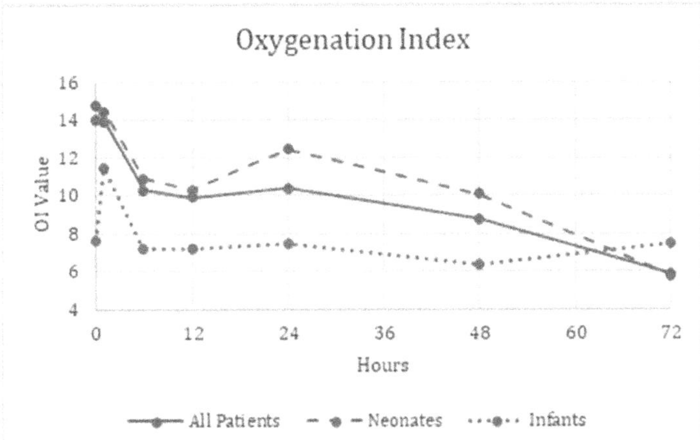

Figure 1. *Cont.*

(d)

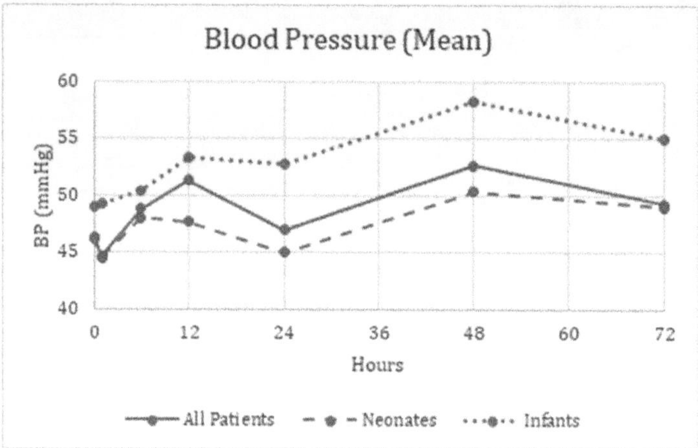

(e)

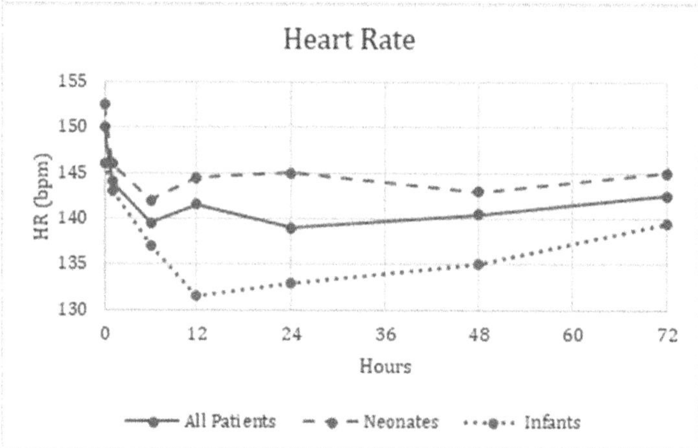

Figure 1. (**a**–**e**) Graphical depiction of the physiologic parameters measured over time in all patients, neonates and infants.

3.4. Safety and Tolerability Data

There were no significant differences reported in the MAP ($p = 0.34$), mBP ($p = 0.12$), or HR ($p = 0.97$) over the study period, suggesting the safety and tolerability of continuous inhaled iloprost in these patients (Figure 1b,d,e). Supplementary Figure S1b,d,e show similar trends in patients who did not need ECMO.

3.5. Patients Who Received Iloprost <6 h (Excluded from Data Analysis)

Seven patients received iloprost for <6 h; four out of seven patients had acute deterioration prompting ECMO cannulation and iloprost discontinuation within the 6 h time period. Two patients did not have evident improvement in oxygenation or hemodynamics with the test dose and one patient had hypotension with severe sepsis.

3.6. Side Effects

No significant side effects were charted. Note that the usual side effects of headaches seen in older patients could not be documented. There was no significant bronchospasm documented with iloprost administration in any patient or need for bronchodilators during the study period. Due to the gradual weaning protocol and background iNO therapy, no rebound PH was noted in our patients. There were no instances of pulmonary hemorrhage or other bleeding attributed to iloprost in this cohort.

4. Discussion

Inhaled prostanoids like iloprost have several advantages over intravenous prostanoids, including the avoidance of significant ventilation perfusion mismatch, potential attenuation of systemic side effects and bypassing vascular access availability or medication incompatibility issues [11,12,19–21]. Subcutaneous prostanoids have been used in this age group; however, pain issues and pump shortage have recently significantly impacted this mode of delivery in the neonatal unit. Inhaled iloprost has the advantage over inhaled epoprostenol because of its longer half-life and stability [6,8]. This medication is often used as rescue therapy in infants with refractory PH despite maximal iNO. Inhaled iloprost is delivered using a syringe pump attached to the port closest to the endotracheal or tracheostomy tube through the inspiratory portion of the ventilator circuit. This is performed to reduce dead space and prevent crystallization in the tubing. In the current study, we have described the methodology of use of continuous iloprost and studied the safety, tolerability and short-term efficacy of the medication in critically ill neonates and infants in a single-institution NICU with refractory WSPH Group 1 or Group 3 PH.

This is the first case series describing the use of continuous iloprost in a NICU cohort with serial evaluation over a 72 h time period. A recent publication by Colglazier et al. describes the methodology of continuous iloprost, which is very similar to our unit but differs from our study in that they were older patients, and the study described the very early response over 30 min of iloprost delivery. Our study is limited the infant age group (<1 year of age) and those with iloprost therapy > 6 h, thus describing the short-to-medium term use of the medication in patients under 1 year of age. Our side effect profile is similar to their study in that continuous iloprost was not associated with significant bronchospasm or any other significant side effects of prostanoids. All our patients on whom iloprost was started were considered refractory PH, already on 20 PPM of iNO (our maximum dose) and hence, we did not compare the two inhaled medications.

Additionally, patient demographics, clinical characteristics and outcomes were reported and stratified with respect to sex (M/F), age (neonate/infant), clinical characteristics (ECMO/No ECMO) and outcomes (survived/deceased) (Tables 1–4). There are several neonatal studies which have suggested male sex as a risk factor for higher incidence of BPD, developmental lung diseases as well as response to therapy; however, in our limited subset, a significant difference was not noted between male and female patients [22–24]. There were very few statistically significant differences between these stratified groups, suggesting that their impact on the efficacy of iloprost is minimal. Verma et al. recently described the potential for inhaled iloprost as a treatment option for PPHN. The trial included 22 neonates with PPHN on intermittent iloprost who did not respond to iNO alone, of whom 55% were considered responders and 45% non-responders who were placed on ECMO or died [12]. This study was limited to PPHN in the neonatal period, which, when not associated with other disorders, usually resolves in 2–3 weeks. Our study includes a whole range of patients with refractory PH secondary to multiple etiologies in the neonatal and infant age groups.

It is possible that the continuous mode of administration reduces the swings in pulmonary and systemic hemodynamics following medication dosage, providing sustained pulmonary vasodilatory effect and minimizing acute blood pressure variations in this fragile population. Additionally, iloprost has also been successfully used as part of strategies to wean and bridge off ECMO support by specifically targeting PH and therefore reducing right ventricular afterload and improving cardiac output. Other studies have speculated that the addition of iloprost to iNO utilizes both the cyclic adenosine monophosphate and cyclic guanosine monophosphate pathways and provides a synergistic effect [10,25]. Since all of our patients were already on maximal doses of iNO prior to initiation of iloprost therapy, the contribution of a synergistic effect in the improved oxygenation status among our patients cannot be established. It is possible that higher doses of iloprost (5–7.5 mcg/h) may have more sustained improvements in PH but our patient numbers and duration of therapy on higher doses were too small to analyze potential effects. Other available inhaled prostanoids include inhaled treprostinil, which is not possible in ventilated patients, but is an attractive option in the outpatient setting. Additionally, some centers use inhaled epoprostenol, using the same preparation as used in the intravenous route, but there is speculation that this preparation may not be suitable for inhaled administration due to potential inflammatory response in the airways and lung parenchyma induced by components in the formulation of this medication [19–21].

As for all infant and pediatric studies, this study is also limited by small numbers, its retrospective format and lacks placebo controls. These were not possible given the patient population being critically ill and iloprost being administered as a rescue medication for refractory PH. Although rSO2 (NIRS) data were also collected, there were multiple missing values precluding meaningful analysis in the current study. Most infants who were cannulated on veno-arterial ECMO had their inotropes stopped, which would impact the significance of VIS scores, especially for patients who were started on iloprost while on ECMO. Thus, the VIS score was not useful in this study. Additionally, in some infants (especially the seven who received iloprost <6 h), iloprost was started during rapid hemodynamic deterioration while being evaluated for ECMO cannulation and the medication was stopped after cannulation on ECMO by physician preference, limiting longer-term evaluation over time in this group. Iloprost was started in a few patients to reduce PH while bridging off ECMO, but the numbers were not adequate for meaningful analysis. A future protocolized strategy of iloprost use in these patients will provide valuable data.

5. Conclusions

This is the largest study describing the use of continuous inhaled iloprost in critically ill neonates and infants with severe pulmonary hypertension. Inhaled iloprost is safe, well tolerated and appears to improve pulmonary and systemic hemodynamics in critically ill infants with PH who usually face very high mortality. Additionally, inhaled iloprost provides an attractive alternate pathway to administer prostanoids. It may also help stabilize some patients prior to ECMO and has the potential to assist in bridging off ECMO in selected patients. Larger prospective multicenter studies are necessary to study the use of this medication in improving outcomes in the infant and pediatric age groups.

Supplementary Materials: The following supporting information can be downloaded at: https://www.mdpi.com/article/10.3390/children11060703/s1, Figure S1a–e depict changes in FiO_2, mean airway pressure, oxygenation index, mean blood pressure and heart rate in patients who did not need ECMO (continuous lines vs patients who needed ECMO (dotted line). The trends on patients who did not need ECMO are similar to all patients depicted in Figure 1. These values become not relevant once patients are placed on ECMO.

Author Contributions: Conceptualization, U.S.K., A.V.K., V.F. and D.S.; methodology, all authors; software, A.V.K.; validation, U.S.K. and D.S.; formal analysis, A.V.K. and U.S.K.; data curation, A.V.K. and V.F.; writing—original draft preparation, A.V.K., V.F. and U.S.K.; writing—review and editing, all authors; supervision, U.S.K. and D.S. All authors have read and agreed to the published version of the manuscript.

Funding: This research received no external funding.

Institutional Review Board Statement: This study was conducted in accordance with the Declaration of Helsinki, and approved by the Institutional Review Board (or Ethics Committee) Columbia University Institutional Review Board approval number IRB-AAAV0892 (1/8/22-1/8/25) for studies involving humans.

Informed Consent Statement: Patient consent was waived due to the retrospective format of the study.

Data Availability Statement: Data are contained within the article and Supplementary Materials.

Acknowledgments: The authors wish to acknowledge Kausalya R. ITM Business School, Chennai, India, for their statistical guidance. They also acknowledge the Pediatric Pulmonary Hypertension Network (PPHNet) for overall mentorship and guidance in management of children with pulmonary hypertension.

Conflicts of Interest: All the authors declare no conflicts of interest.

References

1. Cerro, M.J.; Abman, S.; Diaz, G.; Freudenthal, A.H.; Freudenthal, F.; Harikrishnan, S.; Haworth, S.G.; Ivy, D.; Lopes, A.A.; Raj, J.U.; et al. A consensus approach to the classification of pediatric pulmonary hypertensive vascular disease: Report from the PVRI Pediatric TaskForce, Panama 2011. *Pulm. Circ.* **2011**, *1*, 286–298. [CrossRef] [PubMed]
2. Singh, Y.; Lakshminrusimha, S. Pathophysiology and Management of Persistent Pulmonary Hypertension of the Newborn. *Clin. Perinatol.* **2021**, *48*, 595–618. [CrossRef] [PubMed]
3. Nandula, P.S.; Shah, S.D. Persistent Pulmonary Hypertension of the Newborn. [Updated 2023 Jul 31]. In *StatPearls [Internet]*; StatPearls Publishing: Treasure Island, FL, USA, 2024. Available online: https://www.ncbi.nlm.nih.gov/books/NBK585100/ (accessed on 2 June 2024).
4. Takatsuki, S.; Ivy, D.D. Current challenges in pediatric pulmonary hypertension. *Semin. Respir. Crit. Care Med.* **2013**, *34*, 627–644. [CrossRef]
5. Ivy, D. Pulmonary hypertension in children. *Cardiol. Clin.* **2016**, *34*, 451–472. [CrossRef] [PubMed]
6. Wu, Y.; Liu, H.M.; Gu, L.; Li, Q.W.; Zhu, L. Prostacyclins and pulmonary arterial hypertension in children. *Eur. Rev. Med. Pharmacol. Sci.* **2022**, *26*, 37–45.
7. Barrington, K.J.; Finer, N.; Pennaforte, T.; Altit, G. Nitric oxide for respiratory failure in infants born at or near term. *Cochrane Database Syst. Rev.* **2017**, *2017*, CD000399. [CrossRef]
8. Olschewski, H.; Simonneau, G.; Galiè, N.; Higenbottam, T.; Naeije, R.; Rubin, L.J.; Nikkho, S.; Speich, R.; Hoeper, M.M.; Behr, J.; et al. Inhaled iloprost for severe pulmonary hypertension. *N. Engl. J. Med.* **2002**, *347*, 322–329. [CrossRef]
9. Lakshminrusimha, S. Persistent Pulmonary Hypertension of the Newborn. *NeoReviews* **2015**, *16*, e680–e692. [CrossRef]
10. Colglazier, E.; Ng, A.J.; Parker, C.; Woolsey, D.; Holmes, R.; Dsouza, A.; Becerra, J.; Stevens, L.; Nawaytou, H.; Keller, R.L.; et al. Safety and tolerability of continuous inhaled iloprost in critically ill pediatric pulmonary hypertension patients: A retrospective case series. *Pulm. Circ.* **2023**, *13*, e12289. [CrossRef] [PubMed]
11. Walmrath, D.; Schermuly, R.; Pilch, J.; Grimminger, F.; Seeger, W. Effects of inhaled versus intravenous vasodilators in experimental pulmonary hypertension. *Eur. Respir. J.* **1997**, *10*, 1084–1092. [CrossRef]
12. Limsuwan, A.; Wanitkul, S.; Khosithset, A.; Attanavanich, S.; Samankatiwat, P. Aerosolized iloprost for postoperative pulmonary hypertensive crisis in children with congenital heart disease. *Int. J. Cardiol.* **2008**, *129*, 333–338. [CrossRef]
13. Verma, S.; Lumba, R.; Kazmi, S.H.; Vaz, M.J.; Prakash, S.S.; Bailey, S.M.; Mally, P.V.; Randis, T.M. Effects of Inhaled Iloprost for the Management of Persistent Pulmonary Hypertension of the Newborn. *Am. J. Perinatol.* **2022**, *39*, 1441–1448. [CrossRef] [PubMed]
14. Ivy, D.D.; Doran, A.K.; Smith, K.J.; Mallory GBJr Beghetti, M.; Barst, R.J. Short- and long-term effects of inhaled iloprost therapy in children with pulmonary arterial hypertension. *J. Am. Coll. Cardiol.* **2008**, *51*, 161–169. [CrossRef]
15. Calcaterra, G.; Bassareo, P.P.; Barilla, F.; Martino, F.; Fanos, V.; Fedele, F. Pulmonary hypertension in paediatrics. A feasible approach to bridge the gap between real world and guidelines. *J. Matern. Fetal Neonatal Med.* **2021**, *34*, 3820–3826. [CrossRef]
16. Rimensberger, P.C.; Spahr-Schopfer, I.; Berner, M.; Jaeggi, E.; Kalangos, A.; Friedli, B. Inhaled nitric oxide versus aerosolized iloprost in secondary pulmonary hypertension in children with congenital heart disease: Vasodilator capacity and cellular mechanisms. *Circulation* **2001**, *103*, 544–548. [CrossRef]
17. Hari Gopal, S.; Toy, C.L.; Hanna, M.; Furtun, B.Y.; Hagan, J.L.; Nassr, A.A.; Fernandes, C.J.; Keswani, S.; Gowda, S.H. Inotropic score and vasoactive inotropic score as predictors of outcomes in congenital diaphragmatic hernia: A single center retrospective study. *Front. Pediatr.* **2023**, *11*, 1101546. [CrossRef] [PubMed] [PubMed Central]
18. Belletti, A.; Lerose, C.C.; Zangrillo, A.; Landoni, G. Vasoactive-inotropic score: Evolution, clinical utility, and pitfalls. *J. Cardiothorac. Vasc. Anesth.* **2021**, *35*, 3067–3077. [CrossRef]
19. Kelly, L.K.; Porta, N.F.M.; Goodman, D.M.; Carroll, C.L.; Steinhorn, R.H. Inhaled prostacyclin for term infants with persistent pulmonary hypertension refractory to inhaled nitric oxide. *J. Pediatr.* **2002**, *141*, 830–832. [CrossRef]
20. De Luca, D.; Zecca, E.; Piastra, M.; Romagnoli, C. Iloprost as 'rescue' therapy for pulmonary hypertension of the neonate. *Paediatr. Anaesth.* **2007**, *17*, 394–395. [CrossRef]
21. Berger-Caron, F.; Piedboeuf, B.; Morissette, G.; Simonyan, D.; Chétaille, P.; Pellerin, A.; Hébert, A. Inhaled Epoprostenol for Pulmonary Hypertension Treatment in Neonates: A 12-Year Experience. *Am. J. Perinatol.* **2019**, *36*, 1142–1149. [CrossRef] [PubMed]
22. Debillon, T.; Sentilhes, L.; Kayem, G.; Chevallier, M.; Zeitlin, J.; Baud, O.; Vilotitch, A.; Pierrat, V.; Guellec, I.; Ancel, P.Y.; et al. Risk factors for unfavorable outcome at discharge of newborns with hypoxic-ischemic encephalopathy in the era of hypothermia. *Pediatr. Res.* **2023**, *93*, 1975–1982. [CrossRef] [PubMed]
23. Inkster, A.M.; Fernández-Boyano, I.; Robinson, W.P. Sex Differences Are Here to Stay: Relevance to Prenatal Care. *J. Clin. Med.* **2021**, *10*, 3000. [CrossRef] [PubMed] [PubMed Central]

24. Albert, R.; Lee, A.; Lingappan, K. Response to Therapeutic Interventions in the NICU: Role of Sex as a Biological Variable. *Neoreviews* **2023**, *24*, e797–e805. [CrossRef] [PubMed]
25. Zaccolo, M.; Movsesian, M.A. cAMP and cGMP signaling Cross Talk. *Circ. Res.* **2007**, *100*, 1569–1578. [CrossRef]

children

MDPI

Article

Prevalence of High Blood Pressure in Pediatric Patients with Sleep-Disordered Breathing, Reversibility after Treatment: The KIDS TRIAL Study Protocol

María Castillo-García [1], Esther Solano-Pérez [1], Sofía Romero-Peralta [1], María Esther Viejo-Ayuso [1,2], Laura Silgado-Martínez [1], Leticia Álvarez-Balado [1], Rosa Mediano San Andrés [1], Pilar Resano-Barrio [1], Francisco García-Rio [2,3], Irene Cano-Pumarega [2,4], Manuel Sánchez-de-la-Torre [2,5,6], Alfonso Ortigado [7,8], Ana López-Dueñas [7], Laura Fidalgo [7], Ángel Rodríguez [9], Olga Mediano [1,2,8,*] and Spanish Sleep Network [†]

1 Sleep Unit, Pneumology Department, Hospital Universitario de Guadalajara, 19002 Guadalajara, Spain
2 Centro de Investigación Biomédica en Red de Enfermedades Respiratorias (CIBERES), 28029 Madrid, Spain
3 Pneumology Department, Hospital Universitario La Paz, IdiPAZ, 28046 Madrid, Spain
4 Sleep Unit, Pneumology Department, Hospital Universitario Ramón y Cajal, Instituto Ramón y Cajal de Investigación Sanitaria (IRYCIS), 28034 Madrid, Spain
5 Precision Medicine Group in Chronic Diseases, Respiratory Department, Hospital Universitario Arnau de Vilanova y Santa María, 25198 Lleida, Spain
6 Department of Nursing and Physiotherapy, Faculty of Nursing and Physiotherapy, Universidad de Lleida, IRBLleida, 25002 Lleida, Spain
7 Paediatric Department, Hospital Universitario de Guadalajara, 19002 Guadalajara, Spain
8 Medicine Department, Universidad de Alcalá, 28805 Madrid, Spain
9 Otorhinolaryngology Department, Hospital Universitario de Guadalajara, 19002 Guadalajara, Spain
* Correspondence: olgamediano@hotmail.com; Tel.: +34-949-209-200
† Contributors: Sonia López-Monzoni, Eduardo Laviña-Soriano, Ainhoa Álvarez, Carlos Egea, Genoveva del Río, Fernanda Troncoso, Carolina Díaz and Alejandra Roncero.

Abstract: Current data support an increase in the prevalence of high blood pressure (HBP) in pediatric patients with sleep-disordered breathing (SDB). Adeno-tonsillectomy has been shown to be an effective treatment for most patients. Our objective was to determine the prevalence of HBP in pediatric patients with SDB and the impact of adeno-tonsillectomy with a multicenter, longitudinal, and prospective study that included 286 children referred for suspected SDB. The diagnosis of SDB was established by polysomnography (PSG) and the diagnosis of HBP by 24-h ambulatory blood pressure monitoring (ABPM). In patients without SDB and SDB without treatment indication, these tests were repeated six months after the baseline visit. For patients with medical treatment for SDB, the tests were repeated six months after the treatment initiation. Finally, in patients with surgery indication, ABPM was performed just before surgical treatment and ABPM and PSG six months after the intervention. The study contributes to elucidating the association between SDB and HBP in pediatric patients. Moreover, it contributes to determining if intervention with adeno-tonsillectomy is associated with BP reduction. The results have direct implications for the management of SDB, providing essential information on treatment indications for existing clinical guidelines. NCT03696654.

Keywords: sleep-disordered breathing; high blood pressure; sleep apnea; children; cardiovascular risk; adeno-tonsillectomy

1. Introduction

1.1. Obstructive Sleep Apnea in Children

Obstructive sleep apnea (OSA) is the maximum expression of sleep-disordered breathing (SDB), ranging from simple snoring to OSA [1]. Pediatric OSA is defined as a breathing alteration during sleep, characterized by total (apnea) or partial (hypopnea) obstructions of the upper airway that interfere with normal ventilation and sleep architecture [2]. The severity of OSA is measured by the apnea–hypopnea index (AHI), which shows the number of respiratory events per hour during the sleep. OSA in children is a major public health problem given its high prevalence and its association with relevant consequences, fundamentally in the metabolic, neurocognitive, and cardiovascular spheres [3]. OSA children present nocturnal symptoms such as snoring, nocturnal apneas evidenced by the parents, and enuresis. During the day, the sleep apnea children present with hyperactivity, concentration and memory problems, and somnolence or tiredness [4]. Studies conducted on the prevalence of OSA in children have shown highly variable ratios depending on the population under study, the diagnostic method, and the definitions used. Previous studies have suggested a prevalence of OSA between 1–5% [4,5] in children, with adeno-tonsillar hypertrophy being the most common factor for developing OSA in childhood. A complete polysomnography (PSG) is the diagnostic test for OSA in children that is considered the "gold standard". Additionally, simplified methods have also been validated in the pediatric population [4].

Although being the same disease, OSA is very different between adults and children: the definitions for respiratory event and OSA severity are distinct, diagnosis tools used in adults have less utility in children, and treatment is usually definitive in resolving the events in children and not in adults.

1.2. OSA and Cardiovascular Consequences

During sleep, the patient with OSA is repeatedly subjected to intermittent hypoxia, changes in intrathoracic pressure, and microarousals, which results in the hyperactivity of the sympathetic nervous system, higher oxidative stress, and a proinflammatory and hypercoagulable state [6]. Several studies have suggested that these repeated alterations in each episode of apnea/hypopnea contribute to the development and progression of different cardiovascular diseases, well-documented for high blood pressure (HBP), contributing in these patients to higher mortality and morbidity. In adult patients with OSA, there is an increase in blood pressure (BP) and worse control of it. It has been shown that OSA patients suffer more frequently from a non-dipping pattern and resistant hypertension. The most consistent results relate treatment with continuous positive airway pressure (CPAP) to a reduction in arterial BP [7] and the first signs of atherosclerosis [8]. Randomized clinical trials demonstrate that CPAP treatment reduced blood pressure, was more consistent in resistant hypertension patients and restored the non-dipping pattern [7]. An important aspect is that, to get this effect, a good compliance (better if is more than 6 h per night) is needed [9]. However, the efficacy of CPAP in reducing cardiovascular events has not yet been proven [10,11]. Among the factors that might have influenced this are: (1) the associated cardiovascular illness in OSA adults could be irreversible if treating the disease in adulthood; (2) the presence of cardiovascular risk factors (hypertension, diabetes mellitus, dyslipidemia, etc.) that can act as confounding factors, and (3) the treatment of OSA with CPAP has mainly been suboptimal in this type of clinical trial. For these reasons, the pediatric population constitutes an ideal target group for confirming the impact of OSA on cardiovascular risk prevention: free of established disease and preexisting risk factors, and with effective treatment such as adeno-tonsillectomy. In this way, knowledge of the natural history of the disease would also be facilitated by studying the OSA pediatric population.

1.3. Blood Pressure in SDB in Children

Unlike adults, the diagnosis of HBP in children is based on the normal distribution of BP in healthy children and not on the morbidity and mortality associated with it. In this group, ambulatory BP monitoring (ABPM) during 24 h is more favorable than isolated office BP in predicting morbidity and mortality. ABPM offers advantages over isolated measurements since it allows us to study the variability of BP throughout the circadian cycle and it is more appropriate for predicting organ damage. The 2016 European Guideline for the management of high blood pressure in children [12] continues assuming, as reference values, those provided by the US Task Force [13], in which the values are distributed according to percentiles based on gender, age, and height. However, ABPM is complicated to perform in children, given the difficulty associated with this technique obtaining good quality results.

In children with high BP values, even when these are close to normal levels, it is possible to predict the development of hypertension when they become adults [14], cardiometabolic risk [15], and future coronary disease [16].

Alterations in BP in children have also been associated with OSA, although the evidence is limited. Guilleminault et al. [17] were the first to describe higher BP values among children with OSA. However, Zintzaras et al. [18] published a meta-analysis in 2007 in which they concluded that, until that date, there was insufficient evidence about the relationship between SDB and increased BP. Subsequently, ABPM measurements performed in children with SDB reported elevated systolic and diastolic BP, both during the day and night, independent of obesity status [19,20]. To date, few studies have explored how surgery could improve cardiovascular parameters in children with sleep apnea [21–26]. A significant decrease was observed in systolic and diastolic BP in children with hypertension and OSA after adeno-tonsillectomy compared to non-hypertensive children [27–31].

Additionally, there is limited evidence related to the physiological mechanism implicated in the cardiovascular risk development in children. The study of specific biomarkers, as is troponin T, has been widely studied in adults [32] and could be a good biomarker for children [33].

From the results provided by these studies, it can be deduced that adeno-tonsillectomy could reduce BP in patients with OSA. However, important limitations in most of them (such as small populations, absence of ABPM in most of them, absence of a control group, etc.) make studies in larger population series and with adequate methodology necessary. For this reason, we set ourselves the main objective of evaluating the BP values present in children with SDB and their response to their treatment.

2. Methodology/Design

This article describes the methodology from the registered trial NCT03696654 [34] hypothesis: sleep-disordered breathing increases the prevalence of arterial hypertension in pediatric patients. This hypertension is reversible after treatment.

2.1. Primary Objective

To demonstrate how the presence of sleep-disordered breathing (SDB) is associated with a higher risk of high blood pressure (HBP) in pediatric patients and to confirm that this is reversible with treatment.

2.2. Secondary Objectives

- Establish the relationship between the presence of HBP and the severity of OSA (apnea–hypopnea index—AHI, desaturation index—DI).
- Evaluate the variability along the circadian rhythm of the HBP patterns produced in pediatric patients with SDB.
- Establish the correlation between the diagnosis of HBP measured in the office and by ambulatory control of BP.
- Assess the organic damage produced:
    - Evaluate the manifestation of subclinical organ damage through other markers such as: blood biomarkers (creatinine/glomerular filtration rate), urine (albuminuria/proteinuria), and echocardiography (left ventricular hypertrophy).
    - Establish the pathophysiological mechanisms involved in the HBP/SDB relationship.

2.3. Design and Population

This was a multicenter, longitudinal, prospective study with a control group. A total of 286 children between 4 and 18 years old who were referred prospectively to undergo a sleep study due to suspected SDB were included. The study was directed by the coordinating center (Hospital Universitario de Guadalajara), which was responsible for the study design and patient follow-up. The other participant centers were Hospital Universitario Fundación Jiménez Díaz, Instituto del Sueño, Hospital Universitario Santa Lucía, Hospital San Pedro, and Hospital Universitario de Araba.

2.3.1. Inclusion Criteria

- Approval of the Ethics and Clinical Trials Committee (P02/18).
- Informed consent signed by parents and/or legal guardians.
- Children between 4 and 18 years old evaluated consecutively for suspected SDB.

2.3.2. Exclusion Criteria

- Associated comorbidities: cardiovascular disease (including cardiac malformation), cerebrovascular disease, or unstable severe or exacerbated respiratory disease that preclude the realization of the studies.
- Genetic diseases according to investigator criteria.
- Children with chronic insomnia and/or depressive syndrome.
- Children with malformation syndromes (including craniofacial malformations), Down syndrome, and neuromuscular diseases.
- Previous otorhinolaryngologic surgery and/or CPAP.
- Contraindication for realization of ABPM (arrhythmias, allergy to latex, or coagulation disorders).

Children evaluated for suspected SDB participating in the research study had to meet all the inclusion criteria and none of the exclusion criteria. After informed consent was signed by their parents, the following procedures were developed.

2.4. *Procedures*

Different clinical and anthropometric variables were collected, and the diagnosis of SDB was established by complete PSG and the diagnosis of HBP by taking BP in the office and 24-h ABPM.

2.4.1. Full Polysomnography

PSG was performed according to the criteria of the American Academy of Sleep Studies (AASM 2017). Different signals were recorded, such as nasal flow, snoring, thermistor, thoracic and abdominal movement, transcutaneous capnography, oxygen saturation, heart rate by electrocardiogram, body position, and leg movement. Electroencephalogram recordings will include six electrodes, referred to as contralateral mastoids (A1–A2), adopting the 10–20 rules of international EEG system: two frontal (F3–F4), two central (C3–C4), and two occipital (O1–O2) locations. One ground electrode and another reference electrode (Cz) were included. Two chin electrodes were used to obtain the electromyogram signal and two different electrodes placed above the left and right outer eye cantus were employed to record the electrooculogram (EOG). Apnea is defined as a flow decrease > 90% in two respiratory cycles for obstructive and >20 s or two respiratory cycles accompanied by a desaturation of 3% in central apnea. Hypopnea is defined as a 90–30% flow decrease in two respiratory cycles accompanied by a desaturation greater than 3% or microarousal (AASM 2017). The AHI is defined as the summatory of apneas and hypopneas divided by the sleep time. Based on the results, four groups were created based on the severity of the SDB measured by the AHI: group I: AHI < 3/h; group II: AHI ≥ 3 <5/h; group III: AHI ≥ 5/h <10/h; group IV: AHI ≥ 10/h.

2.4.2. Blood Pressure Measurement

Office BP was measured at the clinic. BP was measured on three occasions, with a pediatric sphygmomanometer validated for pediatric age using the non-dominant arm, the same day as the ABPM (to be used for calibration of the ABPM), and at the post-treatment follow-up visit. The patient needed to be seated for at least 5 min before the BP measures and to remain seated with uncrossed legs and an empty bladder in a quiet environment. Three BP measurements were taken every 3 min, discarding the first one and averaging the last two.

The ABPM study and the BP data collection were done following the recommendations of the European Guide for the management of hypertension in children [12]. Hypertension was considered when systolic blood pressure (SBP) and/or diastolic blood pressure (DBP) were persistently above the 95th percentile according to gender, age, and height and, depending on the distribution of percentiles, the hypertension classification was done. The ABPM was conducted a maximum of fifteen days after the PSG study.

Validated pediatric BP monitoring equipment with sleeves appropriate to the size of the child's arm was used (the size of the cuff to be used is calculated by the average distance between the acromion and the radial head). The device was placed on the non-dominant arm and parents were instructed on how to handle the device (how to turn it off in case of excessive pressure, need to keep the arm still during measurements) and everything related to the test was explained.

For the study of the circadian rhythm pattern in blood BP, a decrease in SBP and DBP of at least 10% (mean BP during the day − mean BP during the night/mean BP during the day × 100) was considered normal.

2.5. Visits and Follow-Up

A full sleep study (PSG) was performed at the sleep unit in the basal visit (Figure 1). The night of the sleep study, parents were provided with the Chervin questionnaire, answering questions (Yes/No) related to the child's behavior both during sleep and while awake. They referred to the habitual behavior of the child in the cardinal or fundamental symptoms of SDB. At the same time, anthropometric measurements were collected by nurses (V1).

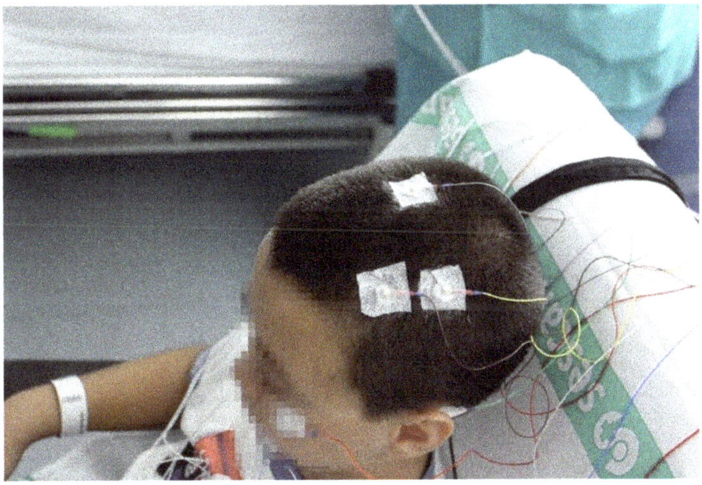

Figure 1. Pediatric polysomnography.

For the HBP study, BP was taken in the office and 24 h-ABPM (V2) was caried out in the following hours (Figure 2).

All patients were offered to participate voluntarily in the determination of subclinical organ damage related to hypertension and the pathophysiological mechanisms involved, which were carried out within a maximum period of one month around the performance of each sleep study (and may coincide with the ABPM study).

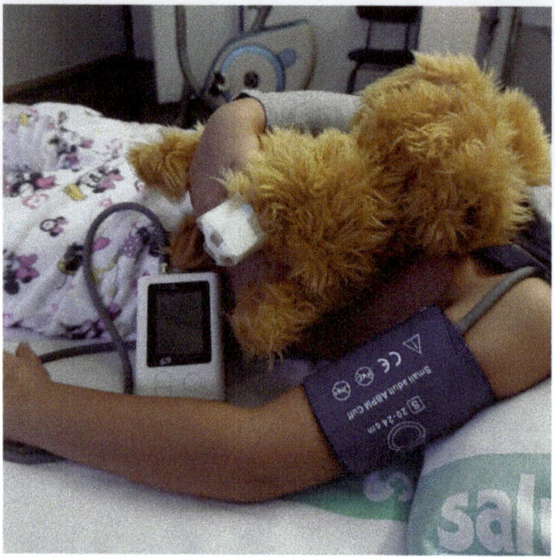

Figure 2. Ambulatory blood pressure monitoring.

Once the sleep study was completed, the therapeutic decision was made in the pediatric clinic based on the criteria established in accordance with the SEPAR sleep-disordered breathing in children consensus (V3) [4].

In order to assess the impact of SDB treatment on BP, measurements were repeated after therapeutic application (V4). In patients who do not require treatment or are referred for medical or orthodontic treatment, the tests were repeated 6 months after the therapeutic decision was made (ABPM, PSG, and organ damage studies, if applicable). In patients referred for adeno-tonsillar surgery, the procedures were repeated just before the intervention (ABPM) and six months after it (ABPM, PSG, and organ damage studies if applicable). Thus, a control group was available without impeding the treatment of any patient and without allowing delays in its application linked to the study (Figure 3).

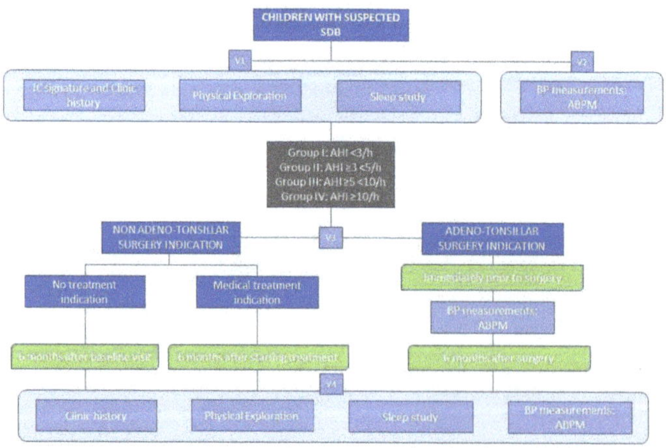

Figure 3. Flow diagram for the study procedure. Abbreviations: SDB, sleep-disordered breathing; IC, informed consent; BP, blood pressure; ABPM, ambulatory blood pressure monitoring; AHI, apnea hypopnea index.

2.6. Study Variables and Data Collection

Data collection was carried out in a database created for this purpose. Here, the variables that participate in the study were registered and stored.

The clinical variables were collected through the Chervin questionnaire, a validate questionnaire usually used in research to identify the presence of SDB in children and to identify important symptoms, including related behavioral disturbances, snoring, and daytime sleepiness [35].

In the physical examination, data of weight, height, body mass index (BMI), neck, hip, and waist circumference, micro-retrognathia (Yes/No), Mallampati (I, II, III, III/IV), tonsillar hypertrophy (I, II, III/IV), adenoid hypertrophy (Yes/No), ogival palate (Yes/No), and bite (III/II/open/asymmetric) were taken.

BMI was corrected for weight and height using established guidelines for converting BMI into percentiles. Based on their BMI, children were classified as: underweight (below the 5th percentile); normal weight (between the 5th and 85th percentile); overweight (between the 85th and 95th percentile); or obese (above the 95th percentile). The sleep study variables included were AHI, DI, minimum saturation, percentage of time below 90% saturation (T90), daytime mean saturation, nighttime mean saturation, sleep efficiency, different sleep states (N1, N2, N3-NREM, and REM), arousal number and index, and leg movement number and index. Central AHI (events with absence of thoracic-abdominal movement) and obstructive AHI (events with presence of thoracic-abdominal movement) were included. Polysomnographic variables were collected through PSG performed during the night period. The PSG was valid if it had >300 valid minutes and >180 min of sleep.

The variability of BP in the circadian rhythm was analyzed by means of ABPM for 24 h, collecting data on SBP and DBP in the office, mean SBP (SBPm), and mean DBP (DBPm) globally, during the day and night, and the non-dipper pattern.

Ambulatory BP measurements were taken every 20 min during the day and every 30 min during the night. A study is considered interpretable when it has at least one reading per hour, 50 readings in 24 h, and 65–75% of the programmed readings. The test can be repeated if it is not valid.

For the determination of subclinical organ damage, the following determinations were included: biomarkers (from blood and urine specimens), electrocardiogram, and thoracic echocardiography (left ventricle hypertrophy—LVH data).

The diagnosis of kidney damage due to HBP is principally made by measuring urine albumin and calculating the glomerular filtration rate (calculated according to blood creatinine, age, and height).

LVH is the most extensively documented marker of organ damage caused by HBP in the pediatric group. Early assessment of LVH in children with HBP is currently recommended as it may facilitate primary prevention of cardiovascular disease. The measure used is the left ventricular mass index (LVMI) (g/m^2), considering LVH when this index is ≥95th percentile (38.6 g/m^2). Between 30–40% of children with HBP had a LVMI above the 95th percentile and in 10–15% this hypertrophy was severe (>51 g/m^2).

2.7. Sample Size Calculation

The sample size was calculated by taking the values reported by Ng DK et al., as a reference [24]. For an alpha risk of 0.05 and beta risk of 0.2 in a bilateral contrast for repeated measures, assuming the standard deviation of the variable in the reference group and with an estimated loss to follow-up of 20%, 286 patients were required to detect a decrease of 2 mmHg in SBPm.

The analysis was carried out with the programs SPSS version 26.0 (IMB SPSS Statistics, CA, USA) and R 2.6.2 (2008, R Foundation for Statistical Computing, Vienna, Austria), accepting a value of $p < 0.05$ as the significance level. The results were presented as mean ± standard deviation or percentage, according to the type of variable. The adjustment of the quantitative variables to the normal distribution was evaluated using the Kolmogorov–Smirnof test. For comparisons between groups, the chi-square or t-Student tests were used.

2.8. Ethical Considerations

This study does not entail relevant risks, except for the discomfort of performing the ABPM study and performing the sleep study control. The ABPM study involves wearing a BP sleeve for 24 h with inflation every 20–30 min. The extraction of biological samples was optional only for those patients who wish to participate in the organ damage sub-study. The study was approved by the Ethics and Clinical Trials Committee (P02/18) and the parents/children signed an informed consent (IC) form. A specific IC was collected for blood and urine samples and biobank storage. Finally, although the study is risk-free, the patients were covered by the general insurance of the National Health System of each participating autonomous community.

3. Relevance of the Study

The management of HBP in pediatric patients continues to be a pending issue in routine clinical practice, even though the presence of high BP levels in children (also values close to normal) has been shown to trigger the progression of hypertension in adults and have a significant association with increased cardiometabolic risk and coronary heart disease in the future.

On the other hand, there is evidence of the involvement of SDB in the presence of HBP levels, relating these SDB with the progression of cardiovascular diseases. Adenotonsillectomy in children with AOS has been recently described to significantly reduce the BP, similarly to adult CPAP treatment. However, the treatment in adults has not been proven to reduce cardiovascular events.

If it is shown that BP increases because of SDB, and that this is reversible after treatment, this would have direct implications for the management of SDB in children and could provide fundamental information on the treatment indications for existing clinical guidelines. Thus, it is important to assess the correlation between SDB in children and future cardiovascular risk, as it could have a relevant impact in clinical practice.

Besides, this information could have enormous relevance for the management of sleep apnea in adults. If the hypothesis of our studies is confirmed, it would imply that the treatment for OSA in children would have a beneficial effect on reducing their future heart attack risk.

Children, unlike adults, are an optimal population because they have no associated risk factors that could act as confounding factors (naïve condition), they have an effective treatment, and they allow for the natural history of the disease to be studied. As a result, they constitute an ideal target for this research, which will also be useful in the management of adults.

For all the above, we advocate that the KIDS TRIAL study constitutes a clear translational study with high potential clinical applicability value.

Author Contributions: Conceptualization, O.M.; methodology, O.M.; validation, O.M. and S.R.-P.; investigation, M.C.-G., E.S.-P., S.R.-P., M.E.V.-A., L.S.-M., L.Á.-B., R.M.S.A., P.R.-B., F.G.-R., I.C.-P., M.S.-d.-l.-T., A.O., L.F., A.L.-D., Á.R., O.M. and Spanish Sleep Network; resources, O.M.; writing—original draft preparation, M.C.-G., E.S.-P., O.M.; writing—review and editing, F.G.-R.; visualization and supervision, O.M. All authors have read and agreed to the published version of the manuscript.

Funding: This work was supported by funds received by the ISCIII (PI18/00565 and PI22/01653), the Spanish Respiratory Society (Sociedad Española de Neumología y Cirugía Torácica- SEPAR) (535-2018 and 1073-2020), unconditioned research grant from Menarini Laboratories and NEUMOMADRID (Sociedad Madrileña de Neumología y Cirugía Torácica).

Institutional Review Board Statement: The study was conducted in accordance with the Declaration of Helsinki and approved by the Ethics and Clinical Trials Committee (P02/18) and was registered as: www.clinicaltrials.gov (first posted on 5 October 2018); NCT03696654.

Informed Consent Statement: Informed consent was obtained from all subjects involved in the study and written informed consent has been obtained from the patients to publish this paper.

Data Availability Statement: Not applicable.

Acknowledgments: We greatly appreciate the participation and cooperation of all children and their parents in the study. We also thank the Spanish Sleep Network for their work on the KIDS TRIAL study.

Conflicts of Interest: The authors declare no conflict of interest.

References

1. Marcus, C.L.; Brooks, L.J.; Ward, S.D.; Draper, K.A.; Gozal, D.; Halbower, A.C.; Jones, J.; Lehmann, C.; Schechter, M.S.; Sheldon, S.; et al. Diagnosis and Management of Childhood Obstructive Sleep Apnea Syndrome. *Pediatrics* **2012**, *130*, e714–e755. [CrossRef] [PubMed]
2. American Thoracic Society. Standards and Indications for Cardiopulmonary Sleep Studies in Children. American Thoracic Society. *Am. J. Respir. Crit. Care Med.* **1996**, *153*, 866–878. [CrossRef] [PubMed]
3. Blechner, M.; Williamson, A.A. Consequences of Obstructive Sleep Apnea in Children. *Curr. Probl. Pediatr. Adolesc. Health Care* **2016**, *46*, 19–26. [CrossRef]
4. Luz Alonso-Álvarez, M.; Canet, T.; Cubell-Alarco, M.; Estivill, E.; Fernández-Julián, E.; Gozal, D.; Jurado-Luque, M.J.; Lluch-Roselló, M.A.; Martínez-Pérez, F.; Merino-Andreu, M.; et al. Documento de Consenso Del Síndrome de Apneas-Hipopneas Durante El Sueño En Niños (Versión Completa). *Arch. Bronconeumol.* **2011**, *47*, 2–18. [CrossRef]
5. Lumeng, J.C.; Chervin, R.D. Epidemiology of Pediatric Obstructive Sleep Apnea. *Proc. Am. Thorac. Soc.* **2008**, *5*, 242–252. [CrossRef]
6. Mediano, O.; González Mangado, N.; Montserrat, J.M.; Alonso-Álvarez, M.L.; Almendros, I.; Alonso-Fernández, A.; Barbé, F.; Borsini, E.; Caballero-Eraso, C.; Cano-Pumarega, I.; et al. Documento Internacional de Consenso Sobre Apnea Obstructiva Del Sueño. *Arch. Bronconeumol.* **2022**, *58*, 52–68. [CrossRef]
7. Martínez-García, M.-A.; Capote, F.; Campos-Rodríguez, F.; Lloberes, P.; Díaz de Atauri, M.J.; Somoza, M.; Masa, J.F.; González, M.; Sacristán, L.; Barbé, F.; et al. Effect of CPAP on Blood Pressure in Patients with Obstructive Sleep Apnea and Resistant Hypertension. *JAMA* **2013**, *310*, 2407. [CrossRef] [PubMed]
8. Lorenzi Filho, G.; Genta, P.R.; Pedrosa, R.P.; Drager, L.F.; Martinez, D. Consequências Cardiovasculares Na SAOS. *J. Bras. Pneumol.* **2010**, *36* (Suppl. 2), 38–42. [CrossRef]
9. Barbé, F.; Durán-Cantolla, J.; Sánchez-de-la-Torre, M.; Martínez-Alonso, M.; Carmona, C.; Barceló, A.; Chiner, E.; Masa, J.F.; Gonzalez, M.; Marín, J.M.; et al. Effect of Continuous Positive Airway Pressure on the Incidence of Hypertension and Cardiovascular Events in Nonsleepy Patients with Obstructive Sleep Apnea: A Randomized Controlled Trial. *JAMA* **2012**, *307*, 2161–2168. [CrossRef]
10. Labarca, G.; Dreyse, J.; Drake, L.; Jorquera, J.; Barbe, F. Efficacy of Continuous Positive Airway Pressure (CPAP) in the Prevention of Cardiovascular Events in Patients with Obstructive Sleep Apnea: Systematic Review and Meta-Analysis. *Sleep Med. Rev.* **2020**, *52*, 101312. [CrossRef]
11. McEvoy, R.D.; Antic, N.A.; Heeley, E.; Luo, Y.; Ou, Q.; Zhang, X.; Mediano, O.; Chen, R.; Drager, L.F.; Liu, Z.; et al. CPAP for Prevention of Cardiovascular Events in Obstructive Sleep Apnea. *N. Engl. J. Med.* **2016**, *375*, 919–931. [CrossRef]
12. Lurbe, E.; Agabiti-Rosei, E.; Cruickshank, J.K.; Dominiczak, A.; Erdine, S.; Hirth, A.; Invitti, C.; Litwin, M.; Mancia, G.; Pall, D.; et al. 2016 European Society of Hypertension Guidelines for the Management of High Blood Pressure in Children and Adolescents. *J. Hypertens.* **2016**, *34*, 1887–1920. [CrossRef] [PubMed]
13. National High Blood Pressure Education Program Working Group on High Blood Pressure in Children and Adolescents. The Fourth Report on the Diagnosis, Evaluation, and Treatment of High Blood Pressure in Children and Adolescents. *Pediatrics* **2004**, *114*, 555–576. [CrossRef]
14. Tirosh, A.; Afek, A.; Rudich, A.; Percik, R.; Gordon, B.; Ayalon, N.; Derazne, E.; Tzur, D.; Gershnabel, D.; Grossman, E.; et al. Progression of Normotensive Adolescents to Hypertensive Adults. *Hypertension* **2010**, *56*, 203–209. [CrossRef] [PubMed]
15. Campana, E.M.G.; Brandão, A.A.; Pozzan, R.; França, M.D.F.; Fonseca, F.L.; Pizzi, O.L.; Magalhães, M.E.C.; de Freitas, E.V.; Brandão, A.P. Pressão Arterial Em Jovens Como Marcador de Risco Cardiovascular. Estudo Do Rio de Janeiro. *Arq. Bras. Cardiol.* **2009**, *93*, 657–665. [CrossRef] [PubMed]
16. Erlingsdottir, A.; Indridason, O.S.; Thorvaldsson, O.; Edvardsson, V.O. Blood Pressure in Children and Target-Organ Damage Later in Life. *Pediatr. Nephrol.* **2010**, *25*, 323–328. [CrossRef]
17. Guilleminault, C.; Eldridge, F.L.; Simmons, F.B.; Dement, W.C. Sleep Apnea in Eight Children. *Pediatrics* **1976**, *58*, 23–30. [CrossRef]
18. Zintzaras, E.; Kaditis, A.G. Sleep-Disordered Breathing and Blood Pressure in Children. *Arch. Pediatr. Adolesc. Med.* **2007**, *161*, 172. [CrossRef]
19. Li, A.M.; Au, C.T.; Sung, R.Y.T.; Ho, C.; Ng, P.C.; Fok, T.F.; Wing, Y.K. Ambulatory Blood Pressure in Children with Obstructive Sleep Apnoea: A Community Based Study. *Thorax* **2008**, *63*, 803–809. [CrossRef] [PubMed]
20. Kang, K.-T.; Chiu, S.-N.; Weng, W.-C.; Lee, P.-L.; Hsu, W.-C. Analysis of 24-Hour Ambulatory Blood Pressure Monitoring in Children with Obstructive Sleep Apnea. *Medicine* **2015**, *94*, e1568. [CrossRef]

21. Amin, R.; Anthony, L.; Somers, V.; Fenchel, M.; McConnell, K.; Jefferies, J.; Willging, P.; Kalra, M.; Daniels, S. Growth Velocity Predicts Recurrence of Sleep-Disordered Breathing 1 Year after Adenotonsillectomy. *Am. J. Respir. Crit. Care Med.* **2008**, *177*, 654–659. [CrossRef] [PubMed]
22. Kuo, Y.-L.; Kang, K.-T.; Chiu, S.-N.; Weng, W.-C.; Lee, P.-L.; Hsu, W.-C. Blood Pressure after Surgery among Obese and Nonobese Children with Obstructive Sleep Apnea. *Otolaryngol.—Head Neck Surg.* **2015**, *152*, 931–940. [CrossRef] [PubMed]
23. Lee, L.-A.; Li, H.-Y.; Lin, Y.-S.; Fang, T.-J.; Huang, Y.-S.; Hsu, J.-F.; Wu, C.-M.; Huang, C.-G. Severity of Childhood Obstructive Sleep Apnea and Hypertension Improved after Adenotonsillectomy. *Otolaryngol.—Head Neck Surg.* **2015**, *152*, 553–560. [CrossRef]
24. Ng, D.K.; Wong, J.C.; Chan, C.; Leung, L.C.K.; Leung, S. Ambulatory Blood Pressure before and after Adenotonsillectomy in Children with Obstructive Sleep Apnea. *Sleep Med.* **2010**, *11*, 721–725. [CrossRef] [PubMed]
25. Apostolidou, M.T.; Alexopoulos, E.I.; Damani, E.; Liakos, N.; Chaidas, K.; Boultadakis, E.; Apostolidis, T.; Gourgoulianis, K.; Kaditis, A.G. Absence of Blood Pressure, Metabolic, and Inflammatory Marker Changes after Adenotonsillectomy for Sleep Apnea in Greek Children. *Pediatr. Pulmonol.* **2008**, *43*, 550–560. [CrossRef]
26. Crisalli, J.A.; McConnell, K.; VanDyke, R.D.; Fenchel, M.C.; Somers, V.K.; Shamszumann, A.; Chini, B.; Daniels, S.R.; Amin, R.S. Baroreflex Sensitivity after Adenotonsillectomy in Children with Obstructive Sleep Apnea during Wakefulness and Sleep. *Sleep* **2012**, *35*, 1335–1343. [CrossRef] [PubMed]
27. Hsu, W.-C.; Kang, K.-T.; Chiu, S.-N.; Weng, W.-C.; Lee, P.-L.; Lin, C.-Y. 24-Hour Ambulatory Blood Pressure after Adenotonsillectomy in Childhood Sleep Apnea. *J. Pediatr.* **2018**, *199*, 112–117. [CrossRef]
28. Kang, K.; Chiu, S.; Weng, W.; Lee, P.; Hsu, W. Ambulatory Blood Pressure Variability after Adenotonsillectomy in Childhood Sleep Apnea. *Laryngoscope* **2022**, *132*, 2491–2497. [CrossRef] [PubMed]
29. Kang, K.-T.; Chiu, S.-N.; Lin, C.-Y.; Weng, W.-C.; Lee, P.-L.; Hsu, W.-C. Trajectory of Ambulatory Blood Pressure after Adenotonsillectomy in Children with Obstructive Sleep Apnea: Comparison at Three- and Six-Month Follow-Up. *Sleep Med.* **2020**, *65*, 127–133. [CrossRef]
30. Kang, K.-T.; Chiu, S.-N.; Lin, C.-Y.; Weng, W.-C.; Lee, P.-L.; Hsu, W.-C. Effect of Adenotonsillectomy on Ambulatory Blood Pressure in Pediatric Obstructive Sleep Apnea: 6-Month Follow-up Study. *Otolaryngol.—Head Neck Surg.* **2019**, *160*, 911–921. [CrossRef]
31. Lee, C.-H.; Kang, K.-T.; Chiu, S.-N.; Chang, I.-S.; Weng, W.-C.; Lee, P.-L.; Hsu, W.-C. Association of Adenotonsillectomy with Blood Pressure among Hypertensive and Nonhypertensive Children with Obstructive Sleep Apnea. *JAMA Otolaryngol.—Head Neck Surg.* **2018**, *144*, 300. [CrossRef] [PubMed]
32. Sánchez-de-la-Torre, A.; Soler, X.; Barbé, F.; Florés, M.; Maisel, A.; Malhotra, A.; Rue, M.; Bertran, S.; Aldomá, A.; Worner, F.; et al. Cardiac Troponin Values in Patients with Acute Coronary Syndrome and Sleep Apnea. *Chest* **2018**, *153*, 329–338. [CrossRef] [PubMed]
33. Duchnowski, P.; Hryniewiecki, T.; Koźma, M.; Mariusz, K.; Piotr, S. High-Sensitivity Troponin T Is a Prognostic Marker of Hemodynamic Instability in Patients Undergoing Valve Surgery. *Biomark. Med.* **2018**, *12*, 1303–1309. [CrossRef] [PubMed]
34. ClinicalTrial.gov. Available online: https://clinicaltrials.gov/ct2/show/record/NCT03696654 (accessed on 20 November 2022).
35. Chervin, R.D.; Hedger, K.; Dillon, J.E.; Pituch, K.J. Pediatric Sleep Questionnaire (PSQ): Validity and Reliability of Scales for Sleep-Disordered Breathing, Snoring, Sleepiness, and Behavioral Problems. *Sleep Med.* **2000**, *1*, 21–32. [CrossRef] [PubMed]

children

MDPI

Article

PICU Survivorship: Factors Affecting Feasibility and Cohort Retention in a Long-Term Outcomes Study

Sarah A. Sobotka [1,*], Emma J. Lynch [1], Ayesha V. Dholakia [2], Anoop Mayampurath [3] and Neethi P. Pinto [4]

1 Section of Developmental and Behavioral Pediatrics, Department of Pediatrics, The University of Chicago, 950 East 61st Street, Suite 207, Chicago, IL 60637, USA; elynch1@peds.bsd.uchicago.edu
2 Department of Pediatrics, Boston Children's Hospital, Boston, MA 02115, USA; ayesha.dholakia@childrens.harvard.edu
3 Department of Biostatistics & Medical Informatics, The University of Wisconsin-Madison, Madison, WI 53705, USA; mayampurath@wisc.edu
4 Division of Critical Care Medicine, Department of Anesthesiology and Critical Medicine, Children's Hospital of Philadelphia, Philadelphia, PA 19104, USA; pintonp@chop.edu
* Correspondence: ssobotka@peds.bsd.uchicago.edu

Abstract: Our understanding of longitudinal outcomes of Pediatric Intensive Care Unit (PICU) survivors is limited by the heterogeneity of follow-up intervals, populations, and outcomes assessed. We sought to demonstrate (1) the feasibility of longitudinal multidimensional outcome assessment and (2) methods to promote cohort retention. The objective of this presented study was to provide details of follow-up methodology in a PICU survivor cohort and not to present the outcomes at long-term follow-up for this cohort. We enrolled 152 children aged 0 to 17 years admitted to the PICU in a prospective longitudinal cohort study. We examined resource utilization, family impact of critical illness, and neurodevelopment using the PICU Outcomes Portfolio (POP) Survey which included a study-specific survey and validated tools: 1. Functional Status Scale, 2. Pediatric Evaluation of Disability Inventory Computer Adaptive Test, 3. Pediatric Quality of Life Inventory, 4. Strengths and Difficulties Questionnaire, and 5. Vanderbilt Assessment Scales for Attention Deficit-Hyperactivity Disorder. POP Survey completion rates were 89%, 78%, and 84% at 1, 3, and 6 months. Follow-up rates at 1, 2, and 3 years were 80%, 55%, and 43%. Implementing a longitudinal multidimensional outcome portfolio for PICU survivors is feasible within an urban, tertiary-care, academic hospital. Our attrition after one year demonstrates the long-term follow-up challenges in this population. Our findings inform ongoing efforts to implement core outcome sets after pediatric critical illness.

Keywords: long-term outcomes; PICU follow-up; neurodevelopment; feasibility; PICU survivors

1. Introduction

Mortality in the pediatric intensive care unit (PICU) has decreased dramatically in recent decades, with a concomitant increase in morbidity, suggesting that mortality alone is no longer a sufficient metric of the long-term impact of critical illness [1–6]. The sequelae of critical illness are diverse; some children exhibit psychological difficulties as a result of traumatic experiences [7–9], while others experience cognitive [10–12] or physical [13] deficits. Post-intensive care syndrome in pediatrics (PICS-p) refers to this constellation of physical, cognitive, emotional, and social health problems facing PICU survivors and their families [14–16]. PICS-p also acknowledges that a child's pre-illness baseline, including pre-existing neurodevelopmental disabilities [17] and other premorbid conditions, may also influence a child's susceptibility to the impact of critical illness [18].

Our understanding of the extent of PICS-p is obscured by the variability in duration of follow-up, patient populations studied, and outcome measures. Importantly, PICU survivors do not have a medical home, distinguishing them from preterm infants or children with congenital heart disease who have dedicated follow-up clinics, potentially placing them at increased risk for loss to follow-up. Studies have assessed outcomes at discrete follow-up intervals [13,19–23], but few have followed children longitudinally. Other studies have been limited to follow-up of survivors with a specific subset of pathophysiology [24–27]. In a scoping review of pediatric critical care medicine literature from 1970–2017, over 360 unique instruments were used to evaluate long-term outcomes [28]. The heterogeneity of these findings limits our understanding of overall PICU survivorship, and in response, there has been increasing attention to the need to develop and implement core outcome sets [29–31] (i.e., standardized sets of outcomes to be measured and reported as a minimum in all effectiveness trials in a specific health area [32–34]). Ultimately, the widespread use of core outcome sets with standardized outcome measures will improve our understanding of PICS-p, allowing for greater comparability across studies.

However, prior to adaption, the factors governing feasibility of implementing core outcome sets must be considered. Among the 407 studies included in a recent scoping review of PICU long-term outcomes studies, enrollment in observational PICU survivorship studies varied from 61–100%, with even lower enrollment in qualitative studies ranging from 20–90% [28]. Retention at long-term follow-up was also highly variable, ranging from 68–100% [28]. In this prospective, longitudinal study piloting the use of multidimensional outcome measures to understand the frequency and natural history of PICS-p and to underscore the challenges associated with longitudinal follow-up among a heterogeneous group of children who experience critical illness, we also sought to measure changes in healthcare utilization and the familial and socioeconomic impact of critical illness and PICU survivorship. Here, we report our experience with regard to feasibility and cohort retention using a multidimensional outcome portfolio among PICU survivors through 3 years after hospital discharge.

2. Materials and Methods

Patients. Patients were enrolled specifically for this study from the PICU at Comer Children's Hospital at the University of Chicago over 15 months (June 2017–August 2018) to account for the seasonal variation inherent in pediatric critical illness and injury. All children aged 0 to 17 years admitted to the PICU were eligible; parental presence at the bedside was necessary for consent and enrollment. No competing clinical or research follow-up programs were in existence at the time of study enrollment, and this cohort does not overlap with previously published cohorts of the authorship team [4,17,35,36]. Children were excluded if they were under state custody due to the logistical challenges of obtaining consent from the state for participation in a research study as well as potential flux in custodial situations at follow-up intervals. Non-English speakers were excluded because some instruments were only available in English with limited ability for translation during remote (telephone or e-mail) follow-up. Informed consent was obtained in person from parent(s)/guardians (hereafter, referred to as "parent(s)"), and assent was obtained from children aged 12 years or older. The protocol was approved by the Institutional Review Board at the University of Chicago.

Screening Process. The study team screened the PICU census for eligible patients and confirmed with the clinical team whether the parent could be approached for consent to participate (potentially denied or deferred due to patient acuity). The study team attempted to recruit several times throughout the hospital stay to capture parents. Bedside nurses facilitated opportunities for consent by notifying the study team when parents became available.

Measures—Enrollment. Measures were selected from existing validated surveys to capture a broad array of functional and neurodevelopmental outcomes. The study team assessed the Functional Status Scale (FSS) score, a validated measure using a five-point scale in each of six domains (mental, sensory, communication, motor, feeding, and respiratory status) from review of the electronic health record (EHR) or parent interview [37]. Parents completed the other survey instruments intended for caregiver informant report directly: 1. the Healthcare and Neurodevelopmental Profile and Family Impact Survey (Impact

Survey), 2. The Pediatric Evaluation of Disability Inventory Computer Adaptive Test (PEDI-CAT), 3. the Pediatric Quality of Life Inventory (PedsQL), 4. the Strengths and Difficulties Questionnaire (SDQ), and 5. the National Institute for Children's Health Quality Vanderbilt Assessment Scales (Vanderbilt). All survey instruments were administered sequentially in a single survey which comprised our PICU Outcomes Portfolio (POP) survey, except for the PEDI-CAT which was administered on an iPad or over the phone. Full details regarding the scoring of the validated instruments are available elsewhere [38–41].

The Impact Survey, designed by the study investigators, captures patients' baseline health utilization and the family impact of the child's illness. Items were cognitively tested with developmental and behavioral pediatric clinic patients prior to study initiation. The final survey length depended on an individual's responses, but included about 30 questions. The Impact Survey includes modified questions from the National Survey of Children with Special Health Care Needs [42] regarding the child's health (e.g., "What kind of place does your child go to when he/she is sick or you need advice about his/her health?"). In addition, questions capture the child's access to and utilization of neurodevelopmental support services (e.g., "Does your child have an IEP (Individualized Educational Program)?"). Family impact is also assessed (e.g., "Has your child's health conditions caused financial problems for your family?"). Supplementary Table S1.

The PEDI-CAT includes 15 items in each of four domains (daily activities, mobility, social/cognitive, and responsibility) to determine the degree of functioning in each category compared to same-aged peers. Adaptive testing maximizes information gathering while minimizing response burden [38].

The PedsQL is a multidimensional tool intended to quantify health-related quality of life in healthy and ill children up to 18 years of age. The PedsQL consists of 23 items in five domains (physical, psychosocial, emotional, social, and school) [39]. This measure was administered to all parents with versions tailored to the age range of the child: 1–12 months, 13–24 months, 2–4 years, 5–7 years, 8–12 years, or 13–18 years. The population mean for parent-proxy reported 81.3 and standard deviation 15.9 for healthy children [43].

The SDQ is a brief behavioral screening survey to assess pro-social behavior and psychopathology of children and adolescents aged 4–17 years [40]. Normative parent SDQ scores for U.S. children are 0–11 (for low difficulties, 12–15 for medium difficulties, and 16–40 for high difficulties [44].

The Vanderbilt is a tool that parallels signs and symptoms from DSM-IV to help healthcare professionals diagnose ADHD in children [41]. The Vanderbilt was administered to parents of children at least 5 years of age. Normative scores data for total Attention Deficit Hyperactivity Disorder (ADHD) score, ADHD inattentive, ADHD hyperactive, Oppositional Defiant Disorder (ODD), Conduct Disorder, and Anxiety/Depression are 3.4, 1.6, 1.8, 1.1, 0.5, and 0.4, respectively [45].

Data were collected and managed using the Research Electronic Data Capture (REDCap) tool [46]. Study staff administered all surveys and collected demographic information (name, age, and medical record number) on an iPad Pro (2017).

The EHR was reviewed for demographic characteristics, admission diagnosis, PICU length of stay, hospital length of stay, and vital signs. Clinical data elements were extracted from the Clinical Research Data Warehouse maintained by the Center for Research Informatics at the University of Chicago in order to calculate the severity of illness indices: Pediatric Risk of Mortality (PRISM) [47] and the Pediatric Sequential Organ Failure Assessment Score (pSOFA) [36] scores.

Measures—Discharge. FSS at hospital discharge was again determined from review of the EHR and/or direct interview with the patient's PICU physicians or nurses.

Measures—Follow-up. Parents were contacted either via telephone or e-mail, per stated preference and contact information (1–2 telephone numbers [home and mobile] and an e-mail address) provided at the time of enrollment. No public or private data searches were conducted to obtain contact information. The child's EHR was queried prior to contact to verify that the parent's telephone number or e-mail had not changed and to ensure that the child had not died in the interval since last contact.

During any specific data-collection period, the study team determined, a priori, that 5 telephone calls within 1 month were reasonable and not intrusive. Parents were contacted at subsequent follow-up intervals even if they had not completed follow-up from the preceding interval. Parents received a 20 USD gift card for each completed follow-up, with a total potential incentive of 80 USD throughout the first year of follow-up and an additional 20 USD annually through to the 3-year follow-up.

A subset of the POP survey was completed at each follow-up interval to decrease overall response burden: 1 month (Impact Survey, SDQ), 3 months (Vanderbilt and PEDI-CAT), and 6 months (PedsQL and FSS). All components of the POP survey except for the PEDI-CAT were completed at 1 year after hospital discharge and annually through 3 years after discharge. Investigators anticipated that the time burden associated with reading the PEDI-CAT over the phone (typically self-administered by the participant using an iPad application) would deter participation, and thus re-administration of the PEDI-CAT was deferred until the 3-year follow-up.

Statistical Analyses. The objective of this presented study was to provide details of data acquisition and follow-up in a PICU survivor cohort and not to present the outcomes at long-term follow-up for this cohort. Descriptive statistics were used to characterize the demographic and clinical variables at each follow-up interval. Participant demographic characteristics were compared to the University of Chicago PICU population during the study period. Follow-up and feasibility data were collected and summarized using descriptive statistics. Analyses were performed using R, version 3.6 (R Project for Statistical Computing, Vienna, Austria), with two-sided $p < 0.05$ denoting statistical significance.

3. Results

3.1. Enrollment

A total of 832 hospitalized patients were screened for enrollment (Figure 1). There were 119 (14.3%) patients who did not meet the eligibility criteria. Of the 713 eligible children, a total of 496 patients were not approached: 228 (32%) due to lack of availability of parents at the bedside, 50 (7%) because the clinical team denied the study team the opportunity to approach parents for consent, and 218 (30.6%) were discharged prior to enrollment opportunity. Thus, of the 217 available parents, 70% (152 parents) provided consent to participate and were enrolled.

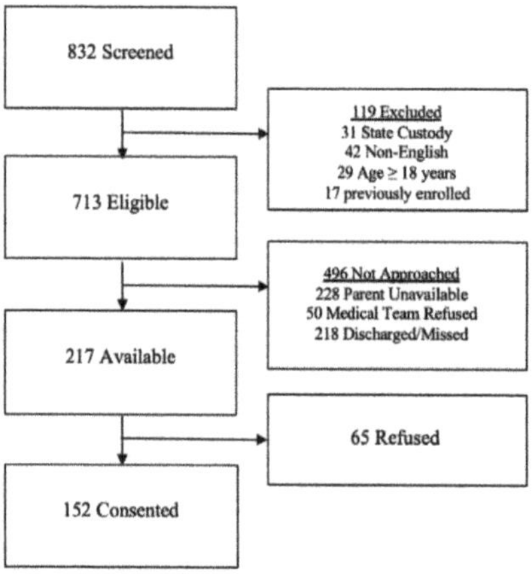

Figure 1. Study enrollment.

3.2. Cohort Characteristics

The University of Chicago Comer Children's Hospital is an urban, academic, tertiary-care center that admits medical and surgical pediatric patients. Demographic and clinical characteristics of the study cohort are presented in Table 1. The median (range) age of the children was 5.2 (0–17) years, and 58.6% were male. Participants were 57.2% African American (n = 87), 33.6% Caucasian (n = 51), 9.2% "Other" (n = 14), and 9.2% Hispanic (n = 14). At the time of study enrollment, our typical patient population was 54.2% male, 59.8% African American, 26.7% White, and 24% surgical patients. Our overall PICU median length of stay was 2.9 days. Our study patients were similar to all patients admitted to the PICU during the study enrollment period with regard to sex, race, ethnicity, severity of illness, and length of stay. Study participants were older than the overall PICU population. (Supplementary Table S1).

Table 1. Demographic and clinical characteristics of study cohort.

Characteristic	Enrollment/Discharge (n = 152)
Age in years, mean (SD)	5.2 (5.2)
Sex, n (%)	
Male	89 (58.6)
Female	63 (41.4)
Race, n (%)	
Black	87 (57.2)
White	51 (33.6)
Other	14 (9.2)
Ethnicity, n (%)	
Hispanic	14 (9.2)
Non-Hispanic	138 (90.8)
Primary Diagnosis, n (%)	
Pulmonary	60 (39.5)
Surgical	33 (21.7)
Neurologic	13 (8.6)
Trauma	12 (7.9)
Infection	11 (7.2)
Other	23 (15.1)
Admission PSOFA, mean (SD) °	4.6 (2.4)
Admission PRISM, mean (SD) °	9.2 (4.5)
Median length of PICU stay °, days (IQR)	3.0 (1.7–8.1)
Median length of Hospital stay °, days (IQR)	4 (3–9)

° admission pSOFA and PRISM calculated as maximum scores within 24 h of PICU admission, hospital LOS calculated as full days during hospitalization encounter; PICU stay determined by time of first and last vital-sign recordings.

Of the enrolled children, the three most common known admission diagnostic categories were pulmonary, surgical, and neurologic (39.5%, 21.7%, and 8.6%, respectively). The median (IQR) PICU length of stay was 3.0 (1.7–8.1) days, and the overall hospital length of stay was 4 (3–9) days. The mean admission pSOFA and PRISM scores were 4.6 (SD 2.4) and 9.2 (SD 4.5). Demographic and clinical characteristics did not vary between patients who did and did not complete follow-up at each time point.

3.3. Cohort Retention and Follow-Up

Of the total 152 patients enrolled, 132 parents (88.6%) completed the 1-month follow-up, 115 (77.7%) completed the 3-month follow-up, 123 (83.1%) completed the 6-month follow-up, and 117 (80.1%) completed the 1-year follow-up. (Figure 2) Of the 152 participants, 122 (80.3%) completed a follow-up for at least 3 of the 4 intervals during the first year of follow-up. At 2 years, 79 (54.5%) children completed the follow-up, and 56 (43.4%)

completed the 3-year follow-up. Three patients died during the study follow-up, and four patients withdrew consent. Sixteen children were excluded from 3-year follow-up because they were ≥18 years of age and parents were no longer eligible to serve as informants.

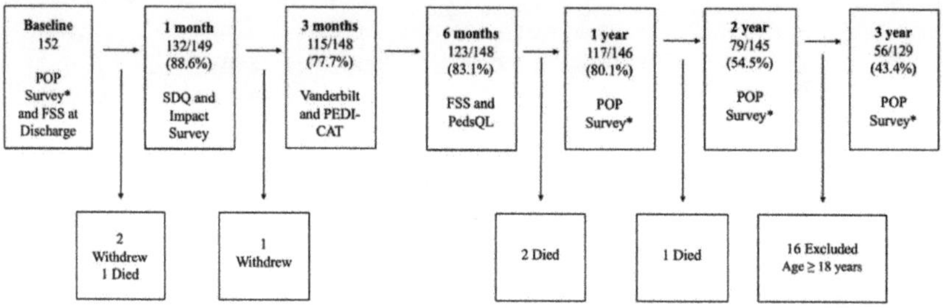

Figure 2. Cohort retention and follow-up among PICU survivors. * POP survey = impact survey, functional status scale (FSS), Pediatric Evaluation of Disability Inventory Computer Adaptive Test (PEDI-CAT), Pediatric Quality of Life Inventory^{TM} (PedsQL), Strengths and Difficulties Questionnaire (SDQ), and Vanderbilt Assessment Scales for Attention Deficit-Hyperactivity Disorder (Vanderbilt); PEDI-CAT was not included at 1- and 2-year follow-up.

3.4. Feasibility Factors

Parents provided their preferred contact method, most often the telephone. E-mail reminders were sent to parents who provided an e-mail address as an alternative contact method. While most parents did not complete their follow-up assessments via e-mail, e-mail correspondence enabled scheduling of telephone follow-ups at a convenient time for parents.

Among the parents who did not complete the follow-up, the median number of follow-up attempts were 6.5 (IQR 4–8) at 1 month, 5 (IQR 4–6) at 3 months, 6 (IQR 2–12) at 6 months, 11 (IQR 6–17.8) at 1 year, 5 (IQR 5–7) at 2 years, and 5 (IQR 5–6) at 3 years. Among the parents who completed the follow-up, the median number of follow-up attempts were 2 (IQR 1–4) at 1 month, 2 (IQR 1–3) at 3 months, 2 (IQR 1–3) at 6 months, 3 (IQR 2–6) at 1 year, 2 (IQR 1–4) at 2 years, and 4 (IQR 3–5) at 3 years. (Table 2). The majority of parents (89–97%) completed the follow-up during weekdays throughout the year. However, study staff attempted follow-ups on weekends with an additional 3–11% of parents. Parents were most often available during daytime hours (7:00 a.m.–4:59 p.m.) with 77–92% of parents completing follow-ups during these hours. Study staff successfully completed follow-ups in the evenings (5:00 p.m.–6:59 a.m.) for 8–24% of parents. The median number of days to completion of a follow-up survey ranged from 9–28 days. However, as many as 19.3% of parents completed their follow-up questions at a subsequent follow-up touchpoint (e.g., completed the 1-month survey at 3 months).

At least five follow-up attempts were made for most children at each interval; however, 13 children had fewer than three attempts documented at one of their follow-up intervals, which may be due to missed opportunities by our study team. With the exception of one child, all were recaptured at later time intervals. We also note that one child with an unusually prolonged hospitalization (>1 year) was inadvertently lost to follow-up because the child's follow-up times did not coincide with the rest of the cohort.

Table 2. Characteristics of successful follow-up attempts.

	Follow-Up Interval					
	1 Month (n = 132)	**3 Months (n = 115)**	**6 Months (n = 123)**	**1 Year (n = 117)**	**2 Years (n = 79)**	**3 Years (n = 56)**
Number of follow-up attempts, median (IQR)	2 (1–4)	2 (1–3)	2 (1–3)	3 (2–6)	2 (1–4)	4 (3–5)
	Day					
Weekday completion, n (%)	127 (96.2)	112 (97.4)	115 (93.5)	104 (88.9)	69 (87.3)	48 (85.7)
Weekend completion, n (%)	5 (3.8)	3 (2.6)	8 (6.5)	13 (11.1)	10 (12.7)	8 (14.3)
	Time *					
Daytime completion, n (%)	116 (89.2)	99 (91.7)	94 (82.4)	88 (76.5)	57 (72.2)	38 (67.9)
Evening completion, n (%)	14 (10.8)	9 (8.3)	20 (17.35)	27 (23.5)	22 (27.8)	18 (32.1)
Days to completion after follow-up eligible, median (IQR)	9 (0–34.3)	26 (10.5–68)	23 (6.5–49)	28 (9–65)	12 (2–28)	38.5 (17.3–124.8)
Completed at later follow-up interval, n (%)	19 (14.5)	21 (19.3)	1 (0.8)	N/A	N/A	N/A

* Time follow-up was not captured for a minority of patients (<10% at all intervals).

4. Discussion

A longitudinal follow-up using a multidimensional PICU core-outcome portfolio is feasible for children and palatable to families discharged from the PICU. Our study has significant findings. Enrollment is the first and greatest hurdle. Consent rates among *available* families were favorable. Retention of this cohort of families for one year was high but there was notable attrition at 2 and 3 years. Our study demonstrates feasibility of implementing a core set of multidimensional outcomes that longitudinally assess the physical, cognitive, educational, social, emotional, behavioral, health-related quality of life, and family impact of pediatric critical illness in a heterogeneous patient population.

Enrollment of parents of PICU patients is challenging; most parents in our urban population were not available for consent and participation. Nearly one-third of eligible parents were not present throughout their child's PICU hospitalization. The lack of parental presence is likely multifactorial due to lack of flexible employment schedules, caregiving responsibilities for other children, transportation barriers, and financial barriers (for food, parking, etc.). Another 30% of children were discharged prior to an approach by the study team, likely due to short stays or discharge at night or on weekends when the study team was not always available (reflecting the aforementioned logistical and socioeconomic challenges). A small percentage of families—7%—were not approached by the study team because of the care team's concerns about suitability for a study focused on long-term outcomes due to the patient's acuity and uncertain prognosis for survival.

While only 21% of all *eligible* families enrolled, the majority of families that were available to the study team agreed to participate. This high consent rate of 70% indicates a subgroup of patients that is willing to participate in studies of long-term follow-up. Our ability to enroll a smaller number of families compared to those who consented, reflecting loss to follow-up, may be explained in part by the demographic and social characteristics associated with risk of poor outcomes. For example, young caregiver age, caregiver language barriers, presence of social supports, transportation challenges, or caregiver intellectual disability are risk factors for adverse PICS-p outcomes [48]. These same factors may inhibit access to care, precluding participation in routine clinical or research-related follow-up.

Our data further reveal that maintenance of a cohesive cohort of 78–89% of these families of PICU survivors during the first year after hospital discharge was possible but necessitates strategic cohort-retention techniques with persistent contact attempts, incentives, flexible modalities, and attention to response burden. Our response rates were comparable to established rates of PICU follow-up at the 3-month follow-up interval. Notably, our response rates at the 1-month, 6-month, and 1-year intervals were more favorable than typical follow-up rates despite the lengthier response burden of the enrollment and 3-month instruments [4,23]. The higher response rates at these three intervals suggest that families were not deterred by the lengthier multidimensional surveys at the preceding intervals. Additionally, parents may have been most willing to participate 1 month after hospital discharge due to the proximity of their PICU experience as compared to subsequent follow-up intervals. Although parents remained highly responsive throughout the 1-year follow-up period, our response rates decreased at 2 and 3 years.

The reasons for our robust follow-up rates and ability to retain the study cohort through 1 year are likely multifactorial. Parents who completed follow-up typically required 2–3 contact attempts, with weekday and daytime hours yielding the highest follow-up rates. Having study staff also available intermittently on weekends and evenings did allow for greater overall cohort retention [49]; notably, the touchpoints during these times were generally brief and not overly burdensome for team members, but occasionally looped in otherwise difficult-to-reach parents. Additionally, our design included multiple attempts to contact parents based on their expressed preferred method of contact, allowed for flexibility regarding scheduling follow-up via telephone or e-mail, and attempted to recapture parents who were "lost to follow-up" at a previous interval. Gift cards for each participation interval may have been an important financial incentive for participation. The majority of parents completed three of the four follow-up assessments over the first year after discharge suggesting that our approach was effective.

Our attention to response burden may have also had a positive impact on our response rates. We informed parents upon enrollment that the outcomes survey was divvied into smaller aliquots except for annual follow-up to proactively manage expectations. We intentionally parsed the study instruments into different intervals to decrease response burden while creating a trajectory for each outcome metric (without a predesignated importance of obtaining certain instruments at specific time intervals). We asked parents to complete any previously missed follow-up instruments at the next follow-up interval, allowing for more complete data and recognizing that parents may differ in availability and willingness to participate.

Our low response rates at 2 and 3 years are not surprising and represent the challenges inherent to long-term remote follow-up. The ability to maintain a meaningful relationship or a relationship without a face-to-face connection is difficult. As more time ensues from PICU discharge to remote follow-up, parents may be less inclined to participate in an activity in which the patient or family does not receive a tangible health benefit (i.e., medical or neurodevelopmental evaluation or therapies). Financial incentive for participation may need to account for this attrition. Future efforts to increase retention rates in PICU follow-up programs would likely benefit from clinician and family education as well as care coordination; education regarding the importance of long-term follow-up and scheduling of these visits prior to discharge have yielded higher rates of neonatal follow-up clinic participation [50].

Our study had important limitations. Because our study design required in-person parent consent and completion of baseline study measures, only 21% of all eligible children were enrolled. We were not able to evaluate the demographic and clinical characteristics of children who did not enroll to understand if they were systematically different from our overall patient population. Our enrollment rates reflect the socioeconomic challenges (single-parent households, competing sibling care demands, inflexible work requirements, poverty, lack of transportation, etc.) that preclude regular parent presence at the bedside. Additionally, we excluded children who were wards of the state or whose parents were primarily non-English speakers due to logistical challenges related to changes in custody after discharge and coordination of interpreter services, parents, and study teams for telephone follow-up. Therefore, our findings may have limited generalizability and may not delineate the additional challenges presented by linguistic barriers. However, our study population was representative of our overall patient population with regard to demographic and clinical characteristics except for older age. Any resultant bias due to an older patient population is unclear, as our EHR does not contain data to determine neurodevelopmental vulnerability. Most parents reported that they had not answered a prior contact attempt because they were busy and did not describe feeling overwhelmed by touchpoints. Directly measuring time burden for parents would provide insight into potential barriers to study completion and inform future work. Semistructured interviews with families to assess the feasibility or perceived burden of participating in longitudinal follow-up studies would further inform efforts to increase recruitment and retention for PICU survivorship studies. Studies indicate that a sense of partnership and family-focused interventions are important facilitators for neonatal follow-up [51,52].

In this manuscript, we report details regarding follow-up methodology and did not present the outcomes at long-term follow-up. In the nascent field of PICU survivorship, providing a methodologic "roadmap" to conduct long-term outcome research is essential. This methodology serves as a starting point for investigators to address the feasibility challenges associated with follow-up studies in a heterogenous population without a common medical home. We did not present methodology and results as a single manuscript because publication page limits would necessitate an abbreviated focus on methodology without the level of detail we were able to provide here.

5. Conclusions

Our results suggest that a multidimensional longitudinal follow-up for a heterogeneous group of children who survive pediatric critical illness is feasible. We identified logistical and resource challenges with enrollment. Frequent attempts to connect with families with flexibility in scheduling remote follow-up, financial incentivization, and minimization of response burden are key elements for retaining a cohort of PICU survivors. Ultimately, understanding the multidimensional scope and trajectories of long-term outcomes facing PICU survivors will allow us to develop and implement interventions that will maximize quality of life and overall functioning for children who experience critical illness.

Supplementary Materials: The following supporting information can be downloaded at: https://www.mdpi.com/article/10.3390/children9071041/s1, Table S1: POP Impact Survey.

Author Contributions: S.A.S. and N.P.P. conceptualized the study, conducted analyses, interpreted results, drafted the manuscript, and orchestrated revision by all coauthors. A.V.D. and E.J.L. assisted with recruitment, data entry, and data analysis. A.M. conducted data analysis. All authors have read and agreed to the published version of the manuscript.

Funding: Sarah Sobotka received support from the Eunice Kennedy Shriver National Institute of Child Health and Human Development (NICHD, K23 HD097276) and the T73 Leadership Education in Neurodevelopmental and Related Disorders Training Program (LEND, T73MC11047). Ayesha Dholakia received support from the University of Chicago Pritzker School of Medicine Summer Research Program and Scholarship and Discovery Program. Anoop Mayampurath received support from the National Heart, Lung, and Blood Institute (K01HL148390). Neethi Pinto received support from The Bucksbaum Institute for Clinical Excellence at The University of Chicago and The University of Chicago Comer Development Board.

Institutional Review Board Statement: The study was approved by the Institutional Review Board of The University of Chicago (protocol code IRB 17-0266 and 18 March 2017).

Informed Consent Statement: Informed consent was obtained from all subjects involved in the study.

Data Availability Statement: The data presented in this study are available on request from the corresponding author. The data are not publicly available.

Acknowledgments: We would like to thank study team members Allison Kniola, Maya Rhine, Maya Krasnow, Nicolas Charron, Khloe Pastore, and Nicole Howard for their contributions to patient recruitment and follow-up. Support for this study was provided by the Department of Pediatrics and the Bucksbaum Institute for Clinical Excellence at The University of Chicago.

Conflicts of Interest: The authors declare no conflict of interest. The funders had no role in the design of the study; in the collection, analyses, or interpretation of data; in the writing of the manuscript, or in the decision to publish the results.

References

1. Namachivayam, P.; Shann, F.; Shekerdemian, L.; Taylor, A.; van Sloten, I.; Delzoppo, C.; Daffey, C.; Butt, W. Three decades of pediatric intensive care: Who was admitted, what happened in intensive care, and what happened afterward. *Pediatr. Crit. Care Med.* **2010**, *11*, 549–555. [CrossRef]
2. Aspesberro, F.; Mangione-Smith, R.; Zimmerman, J.J. Health-related quality of life following pediatric critical illness. *Intensive Care Med.* **2015**, *41*, 1235–1246. [CrossRef]
3. Pollack, M.M.; Holubkov, R.; Funai, T.; Clark, A.; Berger, J.T.; Meert, K.; Newth, C.J.; Shanley, T.; Moler, F.; Carcillo, J.; et al. Pediatric intensive care outcomes: Development of new morbidities during pediatric critical care. *Pediatr. Crit. Care Med.* **2014**, *15*, 821–827. [CrossRef]
4. Pinto, N.P.; Rhinesmith, E.W.; Kim, T.Y.; Ladner, P.H.; Pollack, M.M. Long-Term Function After Pediatric Critical Illness: Results From the Survivor Outcomes Study. *Pediatr. Crit. Care Med.* **2017**, *18*, e122–e130. [CrossRef]
5. Taylor, A.; Butt, W.; Ciardulli, M. The functional outcome and quality of life of children after admission to an intensive care unit. *Intensive Care Med.* **2003**, *29*, 795–800. [CrossRef]
6. Gemke, R.J.; Bonsel, G.J.; van Vught, A.J. Long-term survival and state of health after paediatric intensive care. *Arch. Dis. Child.* **1995**, *73*, 196–201. [CrossRef]
7. Davydow, D.S.; Richardson, L.P.; Zatzick, D.F.; Katon, W.J. Psychiatric morbidity in pediatric critical illness survivors: A comprehensive review of the literature. *Arch. Pediatr. Adolesc. Med.* **2010**, *164*, 377–385. [CrossRef]
8. Bronner, M.B.; Knoester, H.; Bos, A.P.; Last, B.F.; Grootenhuis, M.A. Posttraumatic stress disorder (PTSD) in children after paediatric intensive care treatment compared to children who survived a major fire disaster. *Child. Adolesc. Psychiatry Ment. Health* **2008**, *2*, 9. [CrossRef]
9. Lopes-Junior, L.C.; Rosa, M.; Lima, R.A.G. Psychological and Psychiatric Outcomes Following PICU Admission: A Systematic Review of Cohort Studies. *Pediatr. Crit. Care Med.* **2018**, *19*, e58–e67. [CrossRef]
10. Fiser, D.H.; Tilford, J.M.; Roberson, P.K. Relationship of illness severity and length of stay to functional outcomes in the pediatric intensive care unit: A multi-institutional study. *Crit. Care Med.* **2000**, *28*, 1173–1179. [CrossRef]
11. Bone, M.F.; Feinglass, J.M.; Goodman, D.M. Risk factors for acquiring functional and cognitive disabilities during admission to a PICU*. *Pediatr. Crit. Care Med.* **2014**, *15*, 640–648. [CrossRef]
12. Shein, S.L.; Roth, E.; Pace, E.; Slain, K.N.; Wilson-Costello, D. Long-Term Neurodevelopmental and Functional Outcomes of Normally Developing Children Requiring PICU Care for Bronchiolitis. *J. Pediatr. Intensive Care* **2021**, *10*, 282–288. [CrossRef]
13. Knoester, H.; Bronner, M.B.; Bos, A.P. Surviving pediatric intensive care: Physical outcome after 3 months. *Intensive Care Med.* **2008**, *34*, 1076–1082. [CrossRef]
14. Tang, M.; Xu, M.; Su, S.; Huang, X.; Zhang, S. Post-Intensive Care Syndrome in Children: A Concept Analysis. *J. Pediatr. Nurs.* **2021**, *61*, 417–423. [CrossRef]
15. Manning, J.C.; Pinto, N.P.; Rennick, J.E.; Colville, G.; Curley, M.A.Q. Conceptualizing Post Intensive Care Syndrome in Children-The PICS-p Framework. *Pediatr. Crit. Care Med.* **2018**, *19*, 298–300. [CrossRef]
16. Herrup, E.A.; Wieczorek, B.; Kudchadkar, S.R. Characteristics of postintensive care syndrome in survivors of pediatric critical illness: A systematic review. *World J. Crit. Care Med.* **2017**, *6*, 124–134. [CrossRef]
17. Sobotka, S.A.; Peters, S.; Pinto, N.P. Neurodevelopmental Disorders in the PICU Population. *Clin. Pediatr.* **2018**, *57*, 913–919. [CrossRef]
18. Sobotka, S.A.; Agrawal, R.K.; Msall, M.E. Prolonged Hospital Discharge for Children with Technology Dependency: A Source of Health Care Disparities. *Pediatr. Ann.* **2017**, *46*, e365–e370. [CrossRef]
19. Choong, K.; Al-Harbi, S.; Siu, K.; Wong, K.; Cheng, J.; Baird, B.; Pogorzelski, D.; Timmons, B.; Gorter, J.W.; Thabane, L.; et al. Functional recovery following critical illness in children: The "wee-cover" pilot study. *Pediatr. Crit. Care Med.* **2015**, *16*, 310–318. [CrossRef]
20. Ebrahim, S.; Singh, S.; Hutchison, J.S.; Kulkarni, A.V.; Sananes, R.; Bowman, K.W.; Parshuram, C.S. Adaptive behavior, functional outcomes, and quality of life outcomes of children requiring urgent ICU admission. *Pediatr. Crit. Care Med.* **2013**, *14*, 10–18. [CrossRef]
21. Jones, S.; Rantell, K.; Stevens, K.; Colwell, B.; Ratcliffe, J.R.; Holland, P.; Rowan, K.; Parry, G.J.; United Kingdom Pediatric Intensive Care Outcome Study Group. Outcome at 6 months after admission for pediatric intensive care: A report of a national study of pediatric intensive care units in the United kingdom. *Pediatrics* **2006**, *118*, 2101–2108. [CrossRef]
22. Knoester, H.; Grootenhuis, M.A.; Bos, A.P. Outcome of paediatric intensive care survivors. *Eur. J. Pediatr.* **2007**, *166*, 1119–1128. [CrossRef] [PubMed]
23. Fiser, D.H.; Long, N.; Roberson, P.K.; Hefley, G.; Zolten, K.; Brodie-Fowler, M. Relationship of pediatric overall performance category and pediatric cerebral performance category scores at pediatric intensive care unit discharge with outcome measures collected at hospital discharge and 1- and 6-month follow-up assessments. *Crit. Care Med.* **2000**, *28*, 2616–2620. [CrossRef]

24. Mohsin, S.S.; Haque, A.; Shaikh, A.S.; Bano, S.; Hasan, B.S. Outcome of infants with unrepaired heart disease admitted to the pediatric intensive care unit: Single-center developing country perspective. *Congenit. Heart Dis.* **2014**, *9*, 116–121. [CrossRef]
25. Akhtar, N.; Fadoo, Z.; Panju, S.; Haque, A. Outcome and prognostic factors seen in pediatric oncology patients admitted in PICU of a developing country. *Indian J. Pediatr.* **2011**, *78*, 969–972. [CrossRef]
26. Kamal, H.; Mardini, A.; Aly, B.M. Traumatic brain injury in pediatric age group; predictors of outcome in Pediatric Intensive Care Unit. *Libyan J. Med.* **2007**, *2*, 90–94. [CrossRef]
27. Farris, R.W.; Weiss, N.S.; Zimmerman, J.J. Functional outcomes in pediatric severe sepsis: Further analysis of the researching severe sepsis and organ dysfunction in children: A global perspective trial. *Pediatr. Crit. Care Med.* **2013**, *14*, 835–842. [CrossRef]
28. Maddux, A.B.; Pinto, N.; Fink, E.L.; Hartman, M.E.; Nett, S.; Biagas, K.; Killien, E.Y.; Dervan, L.A.; Christie, L.M.; Luckett, P.M.; et al. Postdischarge Outcome Domains in Pediatric Critical Care and the Instruments Used to Evaluate Them: A Scoping Review. *Crit. Care Med.* **2020**, *48*, e1313–e1321. [CrossRef]
29. Needham, D.M.; Sepulveda, K.A.; Dinglas, V.D.; Chessare, C.M.; Friedman, L.A.; Bingham, C.O., 3rd; Turnbull, A.E. Core Outcome Measures for Clinical Research in Acute Respiratory Failure Survivors. An International Modified Delphi Consensus Study. *Am. J. Respir. Crit. Care Med.* **2017**, *196*, 1122–1130. [CrossRef]
30. Turnbull, A.E.; Sepulveda, K.A.; Dinglas, V.D.; Chessare, C.M.; Bingham, C.O., 3rd; Needham, D.M. Core Domains for Clinical Research in Acute Respiratory Failure Survivors: An International Modified Delphi Consensus Study. *Crit. Care Med.* **2017**, *45*, 1001–1010. [CrossRef]
31. Heneghan, J.A.; Sobotka, S.A.; Hallman, M.; Pinto, N.; Killien, E.Y.; Palumbo, K.; Murphy Salem, S.; Mann, K.; Smith, B.; Steuart, R.; et al. Outcome Measures Following Critical Illness in Children With Disabilities: A Scoping Review. *Front. Pediatr.* **2021**, *9*, 689485. [CrossRef] [PubMed]
32. Williamson, P.R.; Altman, D.G.; Blazeby, J.M.; Clarke, M.; Devane, D.; Gargon, E.; Tugwell, P. Developing core outcome sets for clinical trials: Issues to consider. *Trials* **2012**, *13*, 132. [CrossRef]
33. Fink, E.L.; Maddux, A.B.; Pinto, N.; Sorenson, S.; Notterman, D.; Dean, J.M.; Carcillo, J.A.; Berg, R.A.; Zuppa, A.; Pollack, M.M.; et al. A Core Outcome Set for Pediatric Critical Care. *Crit. Care Med.* **2020**, *48*, 1819–1828. [CrossRef]
34. Topjian, A.A.; Scholefield, B.R.; Pinto, N.P.; Fink, E.L.; Buysse, C.M.P.; Haywood, K.; Maconochie, I.; Nadkarni, V.M.; de Caen, A.; Escalante-Kanashiro, R.; et al. P-COSCA (Pediatric Core Outcome Set for Cardiac Arrest) in Children: An Advisory Statement From the International Liaison Committee on Resuscitation. *Circulation* **2020**, *142*, e246–e261. [CrossRef]
35. Kastner, K.; Pinto, N.; Msall, M.E.; Sobotka, S. PICU Follow-Up: The Impact of Missed School in a Cohort of Children Following PICU Admission. *Crit. Care Explor.* **2019**, *1*, e0033. [CrossRef]
36. Matics, T.J.; Sanchez-Pinto, L.N. Adaptation and Validation of a Pediatric Sequential Organ Failure Assessment Score and Evaluation of the Sepsis-3 Definitions in Critically Ill Children. *JAMA Pediatr.* **2017**, *171*, e172352. [CrossRef]
37. Pollack, M.M.; Holubkov, R.; Glass, P.; Dean, J.M.; Meert, K.L.; Zimmerman, J.; Anand, K.J.; Carcillo, J.; Newth, C.J.; Harrison, R.; et al. Functional Status Scale: New pediatric outcome measure. *Pediatrics* **2009**, *124*, e18–e28. [CrossRef]
38. Dumas, H.M.; Fragala-Pinkham, M.A.; Rosen, E.L.; O'Brien, J.E. Construct validity of the pediatric evaluation of disability inventory computer adaptive test (PEDI-CAT) in children with medical complexity. *Disabil. Rehabil.* **2017**, *39*, 2446–2451. [CrossRef]
39. Varni, J.W.; Seid, M.; Rode, C.A. The PedsQL: Measurement model for the pediatric quality of life inventory. *Med. Care* **1999**, *37*, 126–139. [CrossRef]
40. Goodman, R. Psychometric properties of the strengths and difficulties questionnaire. *J. Am. Acad. Child. Adolesc. Psychiatry* **2001**, *40*, 1337–1345. [CrossRef]
41. Wolraich, M.L.; Lambert, W.; Doffing, M.A.; Bickman, L.; Simmons, T.; Worley, K. Psychometric properties of the Vanderbilt ADHD diagnostic parent rating scale in a referred population. *J. Pediatr. Psychol.* **2003**, *28*, 559–567. [CrossRef] [PubMed]
42. Strickland, B.B.; Jones, J.R.; Newacheck, P.W.; Bethell, C.D.; Blumberg, S.J.; Kogan, M.D. Assessing systems quality in a changing health care environment: The 2009-10 national survey of children with special health care needs. *Matern. Child. Health J.* **2015**, *19*, 353–361. [CrossRef] [PubMed]
43. Varni, J.W.; Burwinkle, T.M.; Seid, M.; Skarr, D. The PedsQL 4.0 as a pediatric population health measure: Feasibility, reliability, and validity. *Ambul. Pediatr.* **2003**, *3*, 329–341. [CrossRef]
44. Bourdon, K.H.; Goodman, R.; Rae, D.S.; Simpson, G.; Koretz, D.S. The Strengths and Difficulties Questionnaire: U.S. normative data and psychometric properties. *J. Am. Acad. Child. Adolesc. Psychiatry* **2005**, *44*, 557–564. [CrossRef]
45. Anderson, N.P.; Feldman, J.A.; Kolko, D.J.; Pilkonis, P.A.; Lindhiem, O. National Norms for the Vanderbilt ADHD Diagnostic Parent Rating Scale in Children. *J Pediatr. Psychol.* **2022**, *47*, 652–661. [CrossRef] [PubMed]
46. Harris, P.A.; Taylor, R.; Thielke, R.; Payne, J.; Gonzalez, N.; Conde, J.G. Research electronic data capture (REDCap)–a metadata-driven methodology and workflow process for providing translational research informatics support. *J. Biomed. Inf.* **2009**, *42*, 377–381. [CrossRef] [PubMed]
47. Pollack, M.M.; Holubkov, R.; Funai, T.; Dean, J.M.; Berger, J.T.; Wessel, D.L.; Meert, K.; Berg, R.A.; Newth, C.J.; Harrison, R.E.; et al. The Pediatric Risk of Mortality Score: Update 2015. *Pediatr Crit. Care Med.* **2016**, *17*, 2–9. [CrossRef]
48. Woodruff, A.G.; Choong, K. Long-Term Outcomes and the Post-Intensive Care Syndrome in Critically Ill Children: A North American Perspective. *Children* **2021**, *8*, 254. [CrossRef]

49. Gildea, M.R.; Moler, F.W.; Page, K.; Meert, K.; Holubkov, R.; Dean, J.M.; Christensen, J.R.; Slomine, B.S. Methods Used to Maximize Follow-Up: Lessons Learned From the Therapeutic Hypothermia After Pediatric Cardiac Arrest Trials. *Pediatr. Crit. Care Med.* **2020**, *21*, 4–11. [CrossRef]
50. Brachio, S.S.; Farkouh-Karoleski, C.; Abreu, A.; Zygmunt, A.; Purugganan, O.; Garey, D. Improving Neonatal Follow-up: A Quality Improvement Study Analyzing In-hospital Interventions and Long-term Show Rates. *Pediatr. Qual. Saf.* **2020**, *5*, e363. [CrossRef]
51. Ballantyne, M.; Benzies, K.; Rosenbaum, P.; Lodha, A. Mothers' and health care providers' perspectives of the barriers and facilitators to attendance at Canadian neonatal follow-up programs. *Child. Care Health Dev.* **2015**, *41*, 722–733. [CrossRef] [PubMed]
52. Ballantyne, M.; Stevens, B.; Guttmann, A.; Willan, A.R.; Rosenbaum, P. Maternal and infant predictors of attendance at Neonatal Follow-Up programmes. *Child. Care Health Dev.* **2014**, *40*, 250–258. [CrossRef] [PubMed]

MDPI AG
Grosspeteranlage 5
4052 Basel
Switzerland
Tel.: +41 61 683 77 34

Children Editorial Office
E-mail: children@mdpi.com
www.mdpi.com/journal/children